AF544996

AEROBICS BASICS

by Karen Liptak

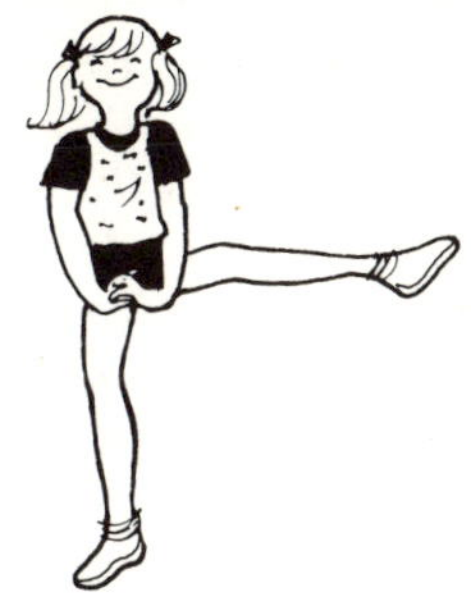

Illustrated by
Janet D'Amato

Photographs by
Susan Warters

Created and Produced by
Arvid Knudsen

PRENTICE-HALL, Inc.
Englewood Cliffs, New Jersey

With many thanks to
ROWENA SINCLAIR-LONG,
Aerobics Teacher Par Excellence,
for her patient and caring choreography

Special thanks to:
Tanya Hubbard, Mary Ann Slate, Lana Wertz, Mary Becker, Teresa Hernandez, Leah Dardis, Ben Sweet, Mariel Celaya, Vanessa Otero, Stevie "G" Romero, Leslie Zepeda, Stephanie R. Reynolds, Stephanie Sylvester from Mrs. Penessa's class at St. Peter and Paul Catholic School in Tucson, Arizona who appear in the photographs of this book.

Other **Sports Basics Books** *in Series*

BASKETBALL BASICS *by Greggory Morris*
RUNNING BASICS *by Carol Lea Benjamin*
DISCO BASICS *by Maxine Polley*
GYMNASTICS BASICS *by John and Mary Jean Traetta*
RACQUETBALL BASICS *by Tony Boccaccio*
FRISBEE DISC BASICS *by Dan Roddick*
SWIMMING BASICS *by Rob Orr and Jane B. Tyler*
HORSEBACK RIDING BASICS *by Dianne Reimer*
SKIING BASICS *by Al Morrozzi*
BASEBALL BASICS *by Jack Lang*
FISHING BASICS *by John Randolph*
FOOTBALL BASICS *by Larry Fox*
SOCCER BASICS *by Alex Yannis*
SAILING BASICS *by Lorna Slocombe*
BICYCLING BASICS *by Tim and Glenda Wilhelm*
BACKPACKING BASICS *by John Randolph*
TENNIS BASICS *by Robert J. LaMarche*
TRACK & FIELD BASICS *by Fred McMane*
HOCKEY BASICS *by Norman MacLean*

Book Design by Arvid Knudsen.

Printed in the United States of America.

Prentice-Hall International, Inc., London
Prentice-Hall of Australia, Pty. Ltd., Sydney
Prentice-Hall Canada, Inc., Toronto
Prentice-Hall of India Private Ltd., New Delhi
Prentice-Hall of Japan, Inc., Tokyo
Prentice-Hall of Southeast Asia Pte. Ltd., Singapore
Whitehall Books Limited, Wellington, New Zealand
Editora Prentice-Hall Do Brasil LTDA., Rio de Janeiro

10 9 8 7 6 5 4 3 2 1

Library of Congress Cataloging in Publication Data

Liptak, Karen.
Aerobics basics.

(Sports basics series)
Includes index.
Summary: Text and illustrations give instructions for a variety of aerobic exercises.
1. Aerobic exercises--Juvenile literature. [1. Aerobic exercises. 2. Exercise] I. D'Amato, Janet, ill. II. Knudsen, Arvid. III. Title. IV. Series.
RA781.15.L56 1983 613.7'1 83-11055
ISBN 0-13-018218-4

CONTENTS

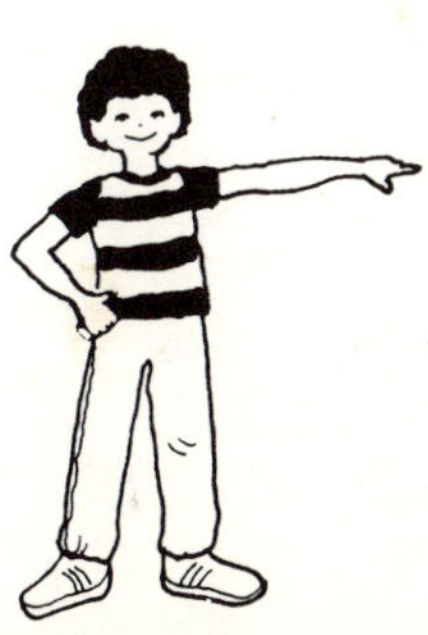

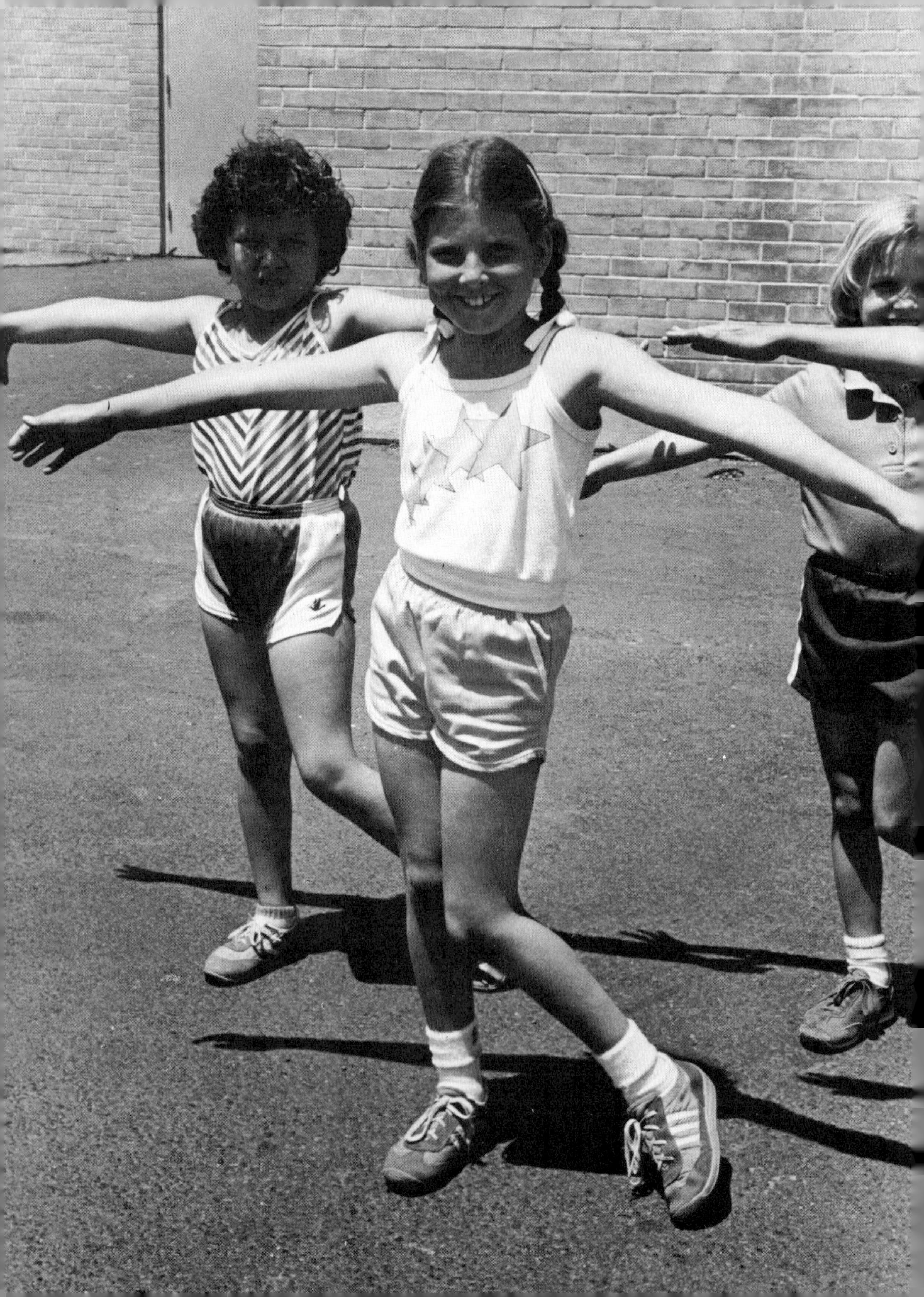

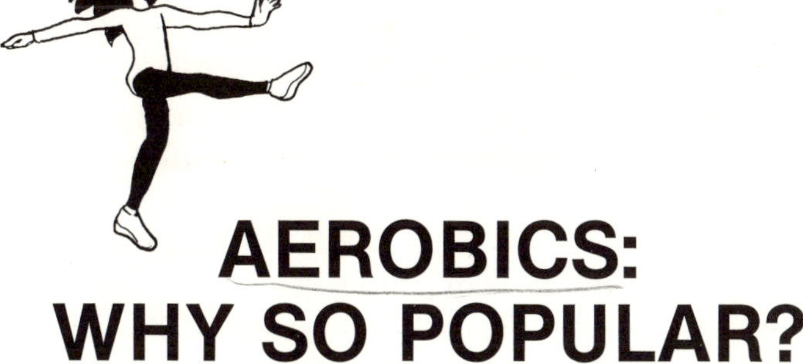

AEROBICS: WHY SO POPULAR?

Chances are you've heard the word aerobics before. In fact, "aerobics fever" seems to have struck our entire country. Superstar Jane Fonda is just one of many famous performers who are avid supporters of the benefits of aerobics in keeping fit and feeling great.

But what, exactly, does "aerobics" mean?

Quite simply, aerobics refers to *a variety of exercises that are done long enough to get your muscles to use a greater amount of oxygen than they normally do.* When this happens, your lung capacity is forced to increase, as your lungs expand to take in and expel more air than is usual for them.

And your heart—one of over 600 muscles in your body—beats more efficiently as it pumps more blood with each beat. This saves your heart a great deal of work, which results in you having more endurance for *all* your activities.

The dramatic effect on your cardiorespiratory system ("cardio" refers to the heart and "respiratory" refers to breathing) is the main benefit of aerobics. But there are many more.

The Benefits of Aerobics

Aerobic activities can help tone up other muscles throughout your body. They can increase your coordination, agility, rhythm, grace, (aerobics teacher Rowena Sinclair-Long calls it your "musicality"), body balance, and stamina.

Aerobics can also improve your feelings of self-confidence and well-being. When you finish an aerobics workout, you *feel* as if you sparkle, and you *look* like you do, as well.

No matter what your favorite sport—football, basketball, figure skating, or disco dancing—your performance is bound to improve faster if your general level of fitness is good. Dr. Jack Wilmore, author of *The Wilmore Fitness Program* and professor of physical education at the University of Arizona, believes that "aerobic fitness is the basic foundation for *any* sport."

Aerobic exercises are also super for helping people slim down and stay in shape. They help you burn off unwanted calories much faster than doing regular everyday activities. And there is medical evidence that the younger you are when you start controlling your weight, the more likely you are to stay in shape for the rest of your life.

Some Popular Aerobic Activities

Jogging, swimming, skating, cross-country skiing, tennis, bicycling, and racketball are some of today's most popular aerobic activities. *But the most rapidly growing aerobic exercise of all is aerobic dancing!*

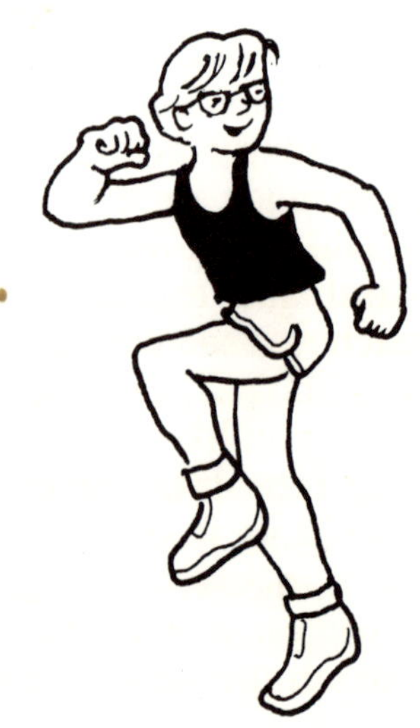

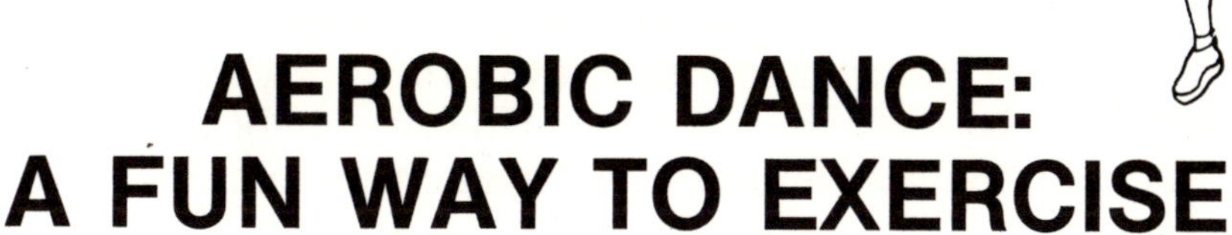

AEROBIC DANCE: A FUN WAY TO EXERCISE

Over the past few years, aerobic dance studios have sprung up all across the country. The reason is simple: *Aerobic dance is not only healthy—it's also great fun!*

When you do aerobic dance routines, you have freedom to do your own thing. Sure there are steps to follow. But you are urged to improvise on them, or even to choreograph your own steps as you move to the music. You don't have to get every step perfect. More important is moving continuously—and enjoying yourself.

Each dance we have presented here leaves plenty of room for your own improvisation. Don't bc afraid to lct go with any of them. Swing your hands as much as you want. Kick as high as you dare. Clap as loud as you can. And sing along if you feel like it.

It's best to get acquainted with one dance at a time by first walking through each step. Learn to do the dance without music. Then when you feel comfortable with the steps, turn on your stereo and start to dance!

For each routine we have suggested certain music that indicates the tempo that best goes with it. But you are free to use any other music you like that has a similar beat. If another song is longer, keep repeating the steps of the dance you are doing. And if another song is shorter, shorten your routine.

We have included six main dance routines for your fun and fitness. And once you get the hang of them, you will be able to mix and match the steps in each to make up original dances.

Before very long you should be able to dance to all your favorite records and tapes. And for a bit of variation, you might turn on your radio and swing and sway, kick and hop, twist and turn to whatever music your local dj has spinning for you. (During commercials jump or jog in place to keep the movement constant to achieve the aerobics effect.)

Basic Aerobics Routine

The six main dance routines in this book range in time from 2:10 minutes to 5:14 minutes. However, to be effective, an aerobics session should last approximately 30 minutes, with 20 minutes devoted to the main dances. To achieve 20 minutes of continuous dancing, you can repeat dances again and again, you can put together your own tape of songs or you can dance to whatever music you have available.

You get the idea by now: Keep moving and the aerobics effect will be yours.

Notice that we have included a variety of *warm-up* and *cool-down stretches.* These are essential parts of every aerobic session. The warm-up stretches will take 5 to 10 minutes before you begin to dance. And the cool-down stretches will take 5 to 10 minutes at the end of your dance session.

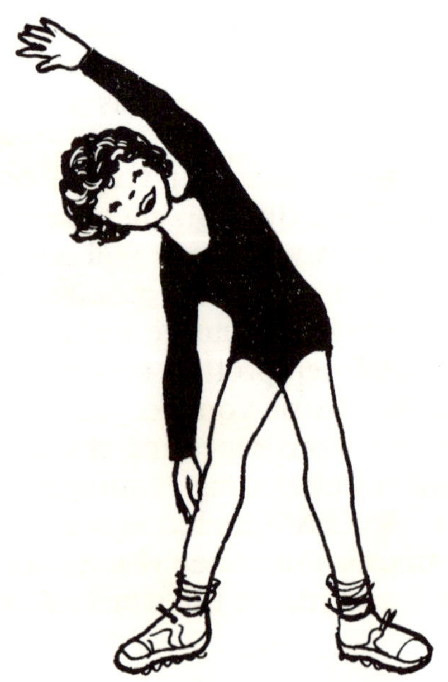

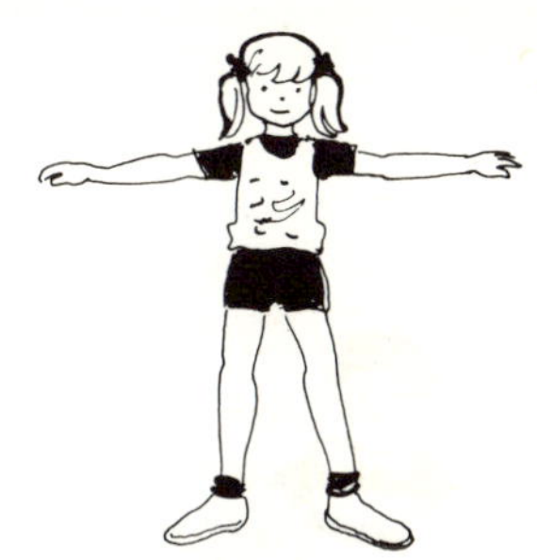

HOW TO START DANCIN'

Time: There is no special time of day when you should do aerobic dancing. Some people enjoy this kind of exercise in the morning. Others, later on in the day. You may want to dance as a break between coming home from school and doing your homework. Or, you may choose to dance as a well-deserved reward after your homework is out of the way.

However, there are two times during the day when it is wise to avoid vigorous activity: right after you eat (you might interfere with your digestion and get cramps) and right before bedtime (you might get too hyped up to fall asleep).

Frequency: Aerobic activities are most effective when they are done at least three times a week. Alternating days (Monday, Wednesday, Friday) is better than exercising on consecutive days, followed by a long stretch of inactivity. And you can substitute other aerobic activities for dance (you might enjoy aerobic dancing twice a week and swimming or tennis once a week).

Place: Choose a well-ventilated area, one that isn't too hot or too cold. The space should give you plenty of room in which to move around freely. If furniture is in the way, perhaps you can move it to one side. A wooden floor or one that is carpeted is best to dance on. (Be wary of unsecured scatter rugs. They could make you trip.)

Clothing: Your aerobics costume should be something loose and comfortable. Leotards, tights, and legwarmers will look stylish, of course, but shorts and T-shirts will do just as well. For your feet, choose a good pair of running shoes. They will help to cushion your whole body against the stresses placed on it by your vigorous aerobic movements.

Caution: Should you feel sick, it is best to rest, rather than force yourself to exercise.

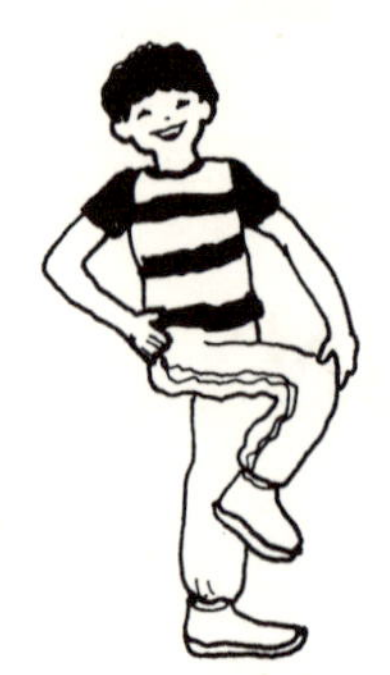

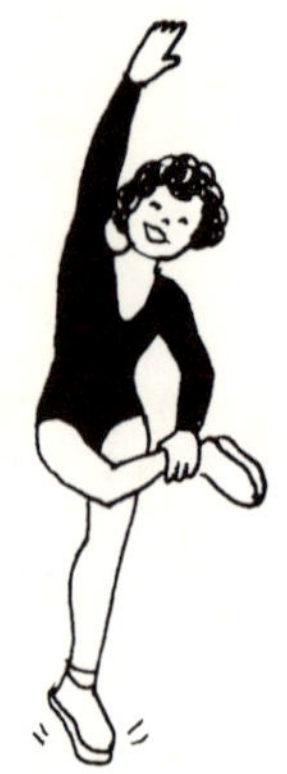

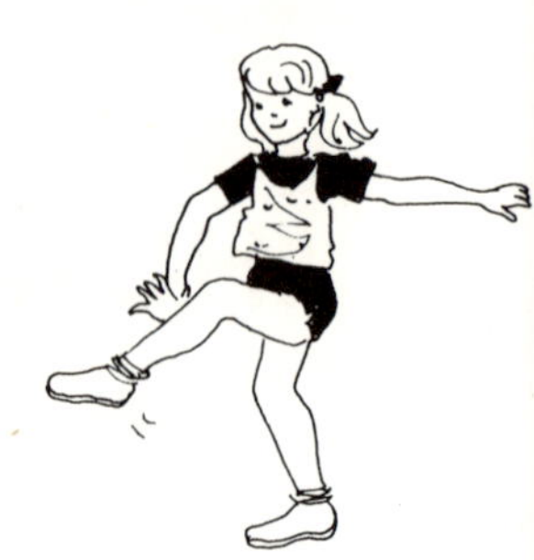

AEROBIC DANCING: A FAMILY AFFAIR

The exciting dance routines we have included in this book are designed for both girls and boys. In fact, aerobic dancing is one activity the whole family can enjoy together. Aerobics teacher Rowena Sinclair-Long, who has choreographed all the dances in *Aerobics Basics*, even teaches a class for mothers and toddlers!

When it comes to aerobic dancing, the whole family can get in the act—the more the merrier!

If you're the type who prefers company when you dance, you might set up a class for your family and friends. You can learn the steps ahead of time and act as the teacher. Or everyone can learn the steps together, right from this book. Once your classmates sample the fun and the good feeling that comes from getting in shape, don't be surprised if aerobic dance classes become a regular event at your home!

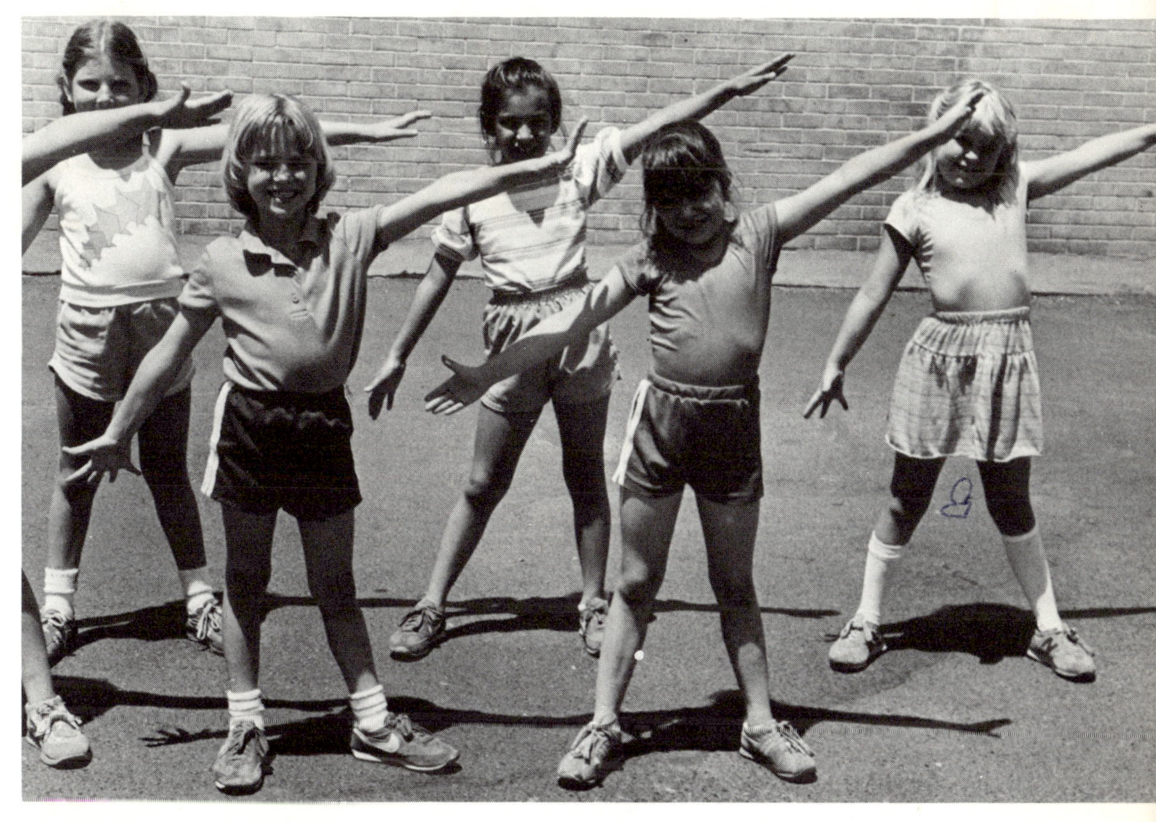

AEROBICS BASICS WARM-UPS

These flexibility exercises will help you to limber up your body for the aerobic dances that lie ahead. The secret to warming up properly is not in how many times you repeat each exercise, but in how long you hold each stretch. Do each of the following warm-up stretches 5 times each. And hold each stretch you do for a slow count of 5 (1000, 2000, 3000, 4000, 5000).

Suggested music: *Let It Be*, by The Beatles
Isn't It Lovely, by Stevie Wonder

WARM-UP STRETCH 1

STANDING STRETCH

A. Stretch right arm over head as you bend body to left.
B. Slide left hand down side of left leg to left knee. Hold.
C. Repeat stretch on right side.

Repeat all 5 times.

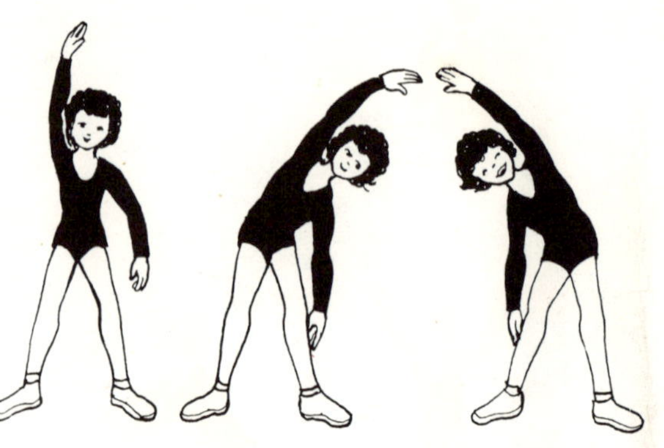

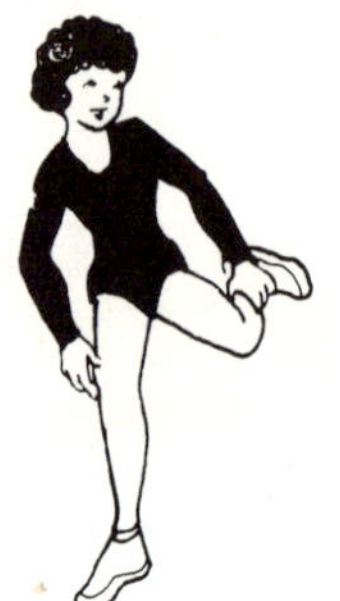

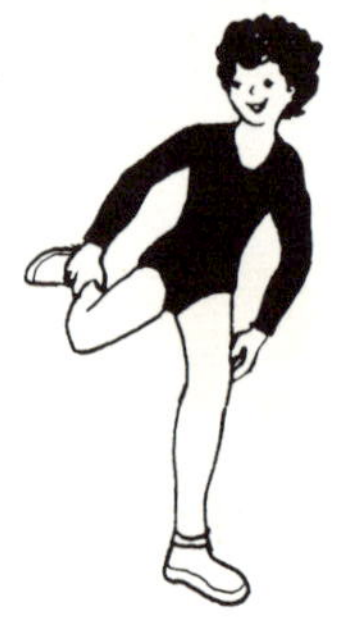

WARM-UP STRETCH 2

PULL-BACK STRETCH

A. Pull left leg back with left hand. (Right hand is on right leg.) Hold.
B. Repeat with right leg.

Repeat both 5 times.

WARM-UP STRETCH 3

WIDE-SEATED STRETCH

A. Sit on floor with knees facing up, legs apart, arms at sides.
B. Slide arms down legs until you can touch lower legs (or toes). Hold.

Repeat 5 times.

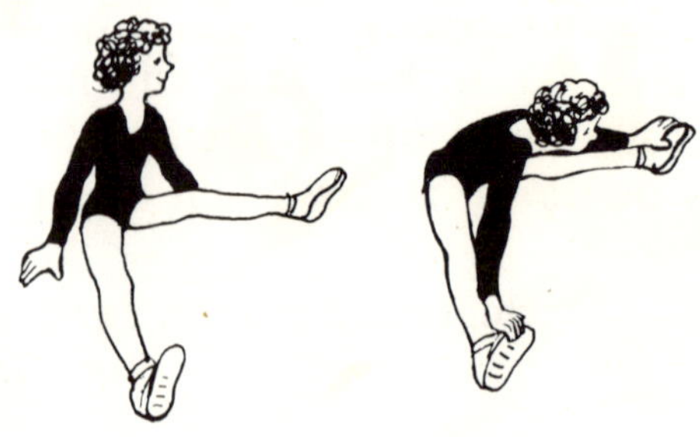

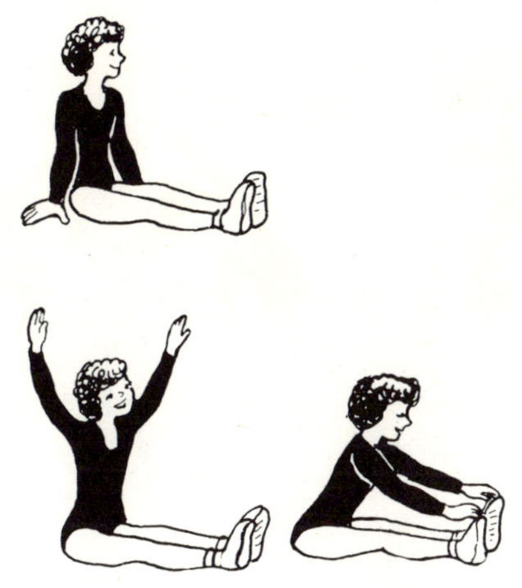

WARM-UP STRETCH 4

STRAIGHT-SEATED STRETCH

A. Sit on floor with legs straight together, arms at sides.
B. Raise arms overhead and stretch forward as far as you can. Hold.
Repeat 5 times.

WARM-UP STRETCH 5

HEEL-LIFT STRETCH

A. Stand with feet slightly apart, hands on hips.
B. Raise heels as high as you can, balancing on toes. Hold.
Repeat 5 times.

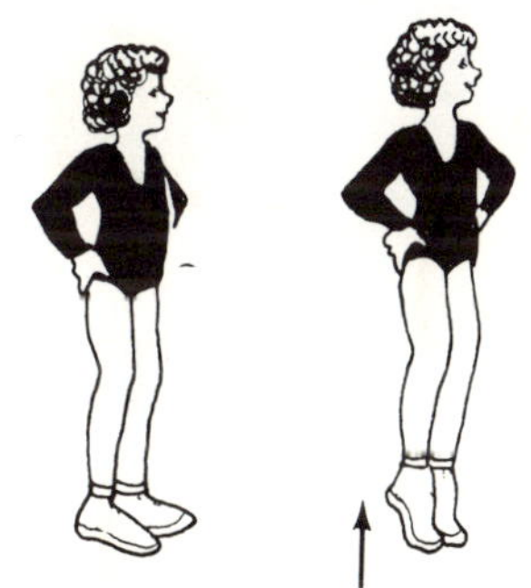

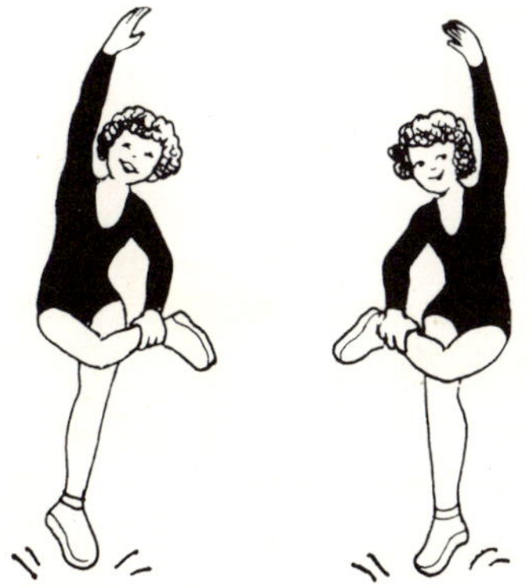

WARM-UP STRETCH 6

HEEL-GRASP STRETCH

A. Grasp right ankle with left hand while right arm is raised. Hop 10 times, then hold.
B. Repeat with opposite side.
Repeat both 5 times.

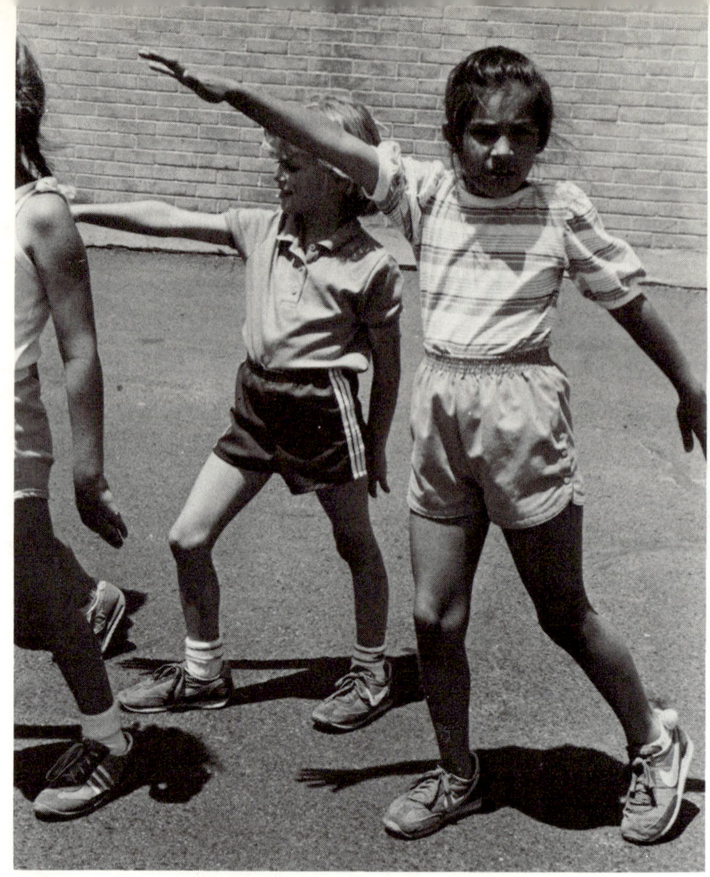

TUCSON TWIST

Here's a fun dance for you! Once you've gotten the steps down pat, you'll find it natural to put in a few "yippees" and "yahoos" as you move to the music. The Tucson Twist goes great with lots of different kinds of country and western music. It's also especially good for boys and girls to dance together.

Suggested music: *The Cowgirl Song* (2:10 minutes), by Moe Bandy and Joe Stampley

Alternate music: *Electric Horseman, Oh, Susanna.*

STEP 1

LUNGES

1. Lunge left, with right leg straight. Right hand is straight out, left hand is on left hip.
2. Lunge right, with left leg straight. Left hand is straight out, right hand is on right hip.
3. Repeat lunges: left, right, left, right, left, right.
4. Hop-twist left, right, left, arms straight out.
5. Repeat lunges: left, right, left, right.

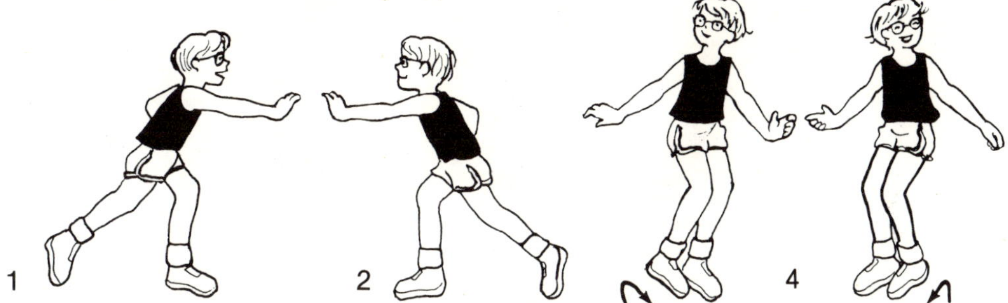

STEP 2

HEEL-TOE

(Face front, hands on hips)

1. Place right heel to side, toes up.
2. Bend right knee so right toes nearly touch left foot.
3. Repeat right heel-toe.
4. Kick with right leg.
5. Step right with left foot, bring feet together.
6. Place left heel to side, toes up.
7. Bend left knee so left toes nearly touch left foot.
8. Repeat left heel-toe.
9. Kick with left leg.
10. Step left with right foot, bring feet together.
11. Repeat right heel-toe, left heel-toe.

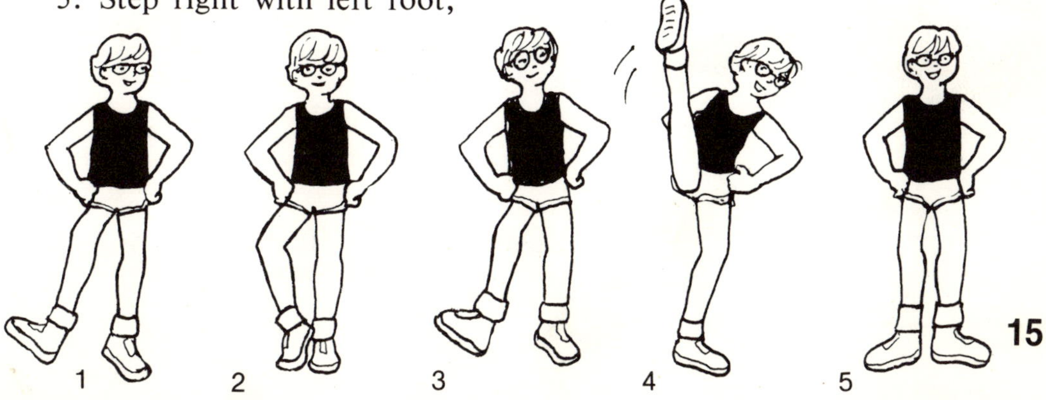

STEP 3

*AST = at same time.

CIRCLE RUN

1. Run in place, moving in a small circle going right.

*AST: Alternate straight arms moving up and down.

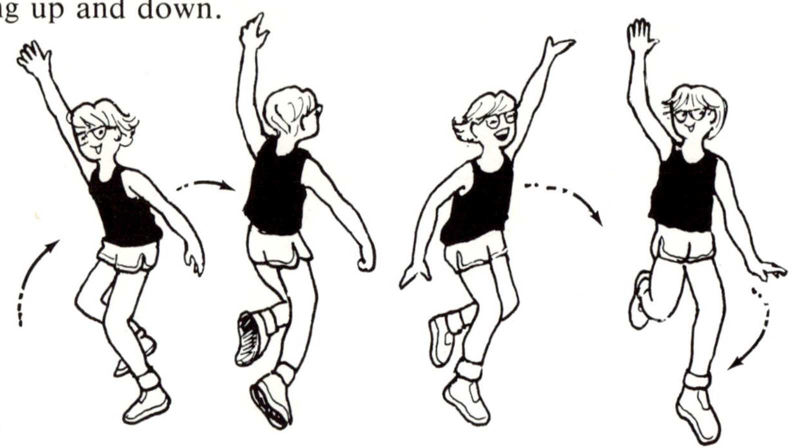

STEP 4

DOSIDO

(Face front)

1. Move back by first skipping on left foot, then right foot, then left, then right.

AST: Bend elbow of opposite arm at chest.

2. Move forward, skipping left, right, left, right.
3. Move back again.
4. Move forward again.

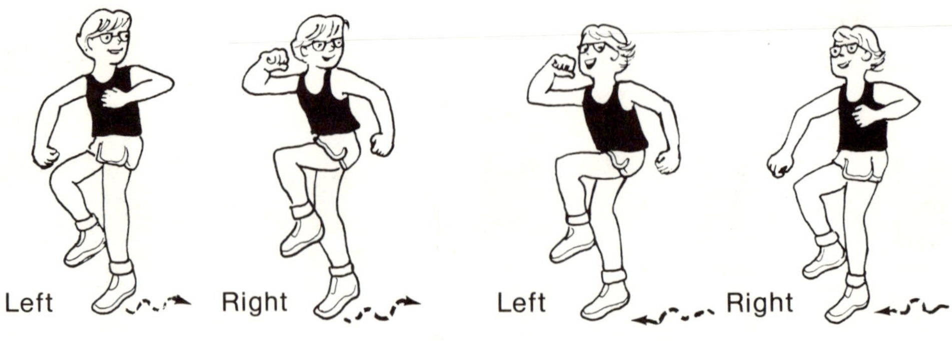

STEP 5

3-WAY CLAPS

1. Jump left and clap hands on thighs.
2. Clap hands together.
3. Jump center and clap hands on thighs.
4. Clap hands together.
5. Jump right and clap hands on thighs.
6. Clap hands together.

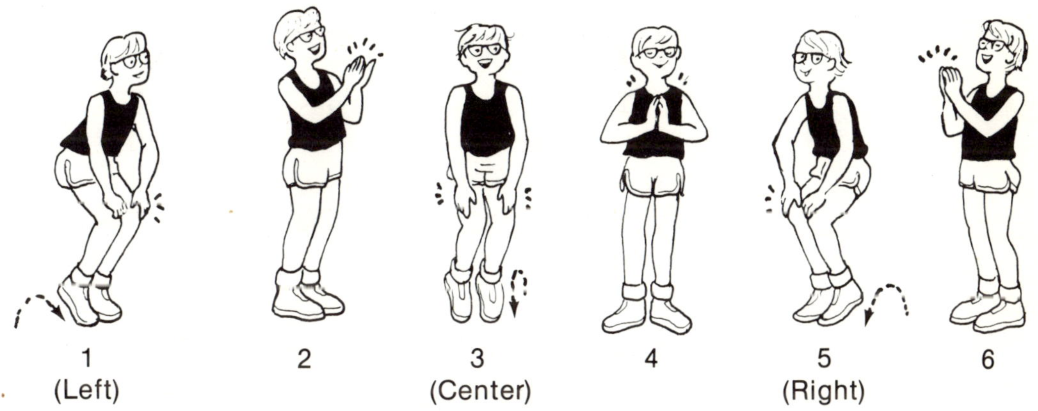

Repeat:
Step 2: Heel-toe, right, left, right, left
Step 3: Circle run
Step 4: Dosido
Step 5: 3-way claps (2 times)
Step 2: Heel-toe (Continue until music ends.)

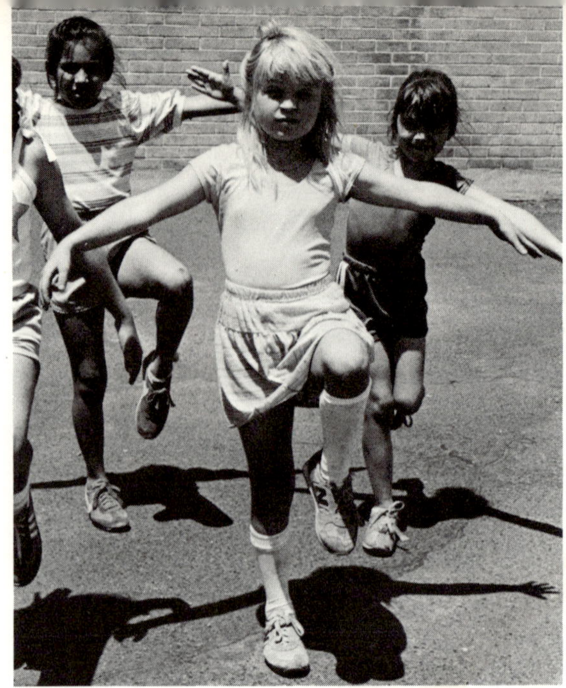

KANSAS CITY KICK

This rhythmic dance has lots of stretching in it for every part of your body. Whether you're living in Kansas City or anywhere else, you'll love kicking up your heels and moving to the music.

Suggested music: *The Smurf* (3:38 minutes), by Tyrone Brunson
Alternate music: *Sunset People, Just Another Man*

INTRODUCTION:

Face front with feet apart and arms at sides, palms face in. Lift right arm, left arm. Lower right arm to side. Lower left arm to side. Lower both arms to legs. Lift both arms up.

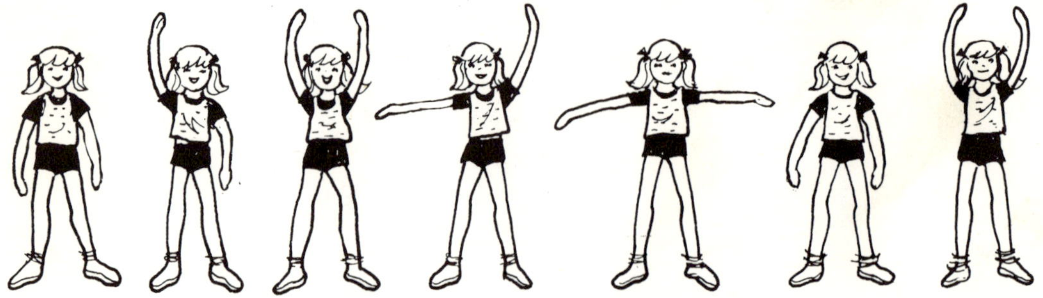

STEP 1

BEND-KICKS

1. Face front, feet apart.
2. Kick right leg across left, touch with left palm.
3. Feet down, hands out.
4. Kick left leg across right, touch with right palm.
5. Feet down, hands out.
6. Kick right leg back. AST: Clap hands.
7. Feet down, hands out.
8. Kick left leg back. AST: Clap hands.
9. Repeat 3 more times.

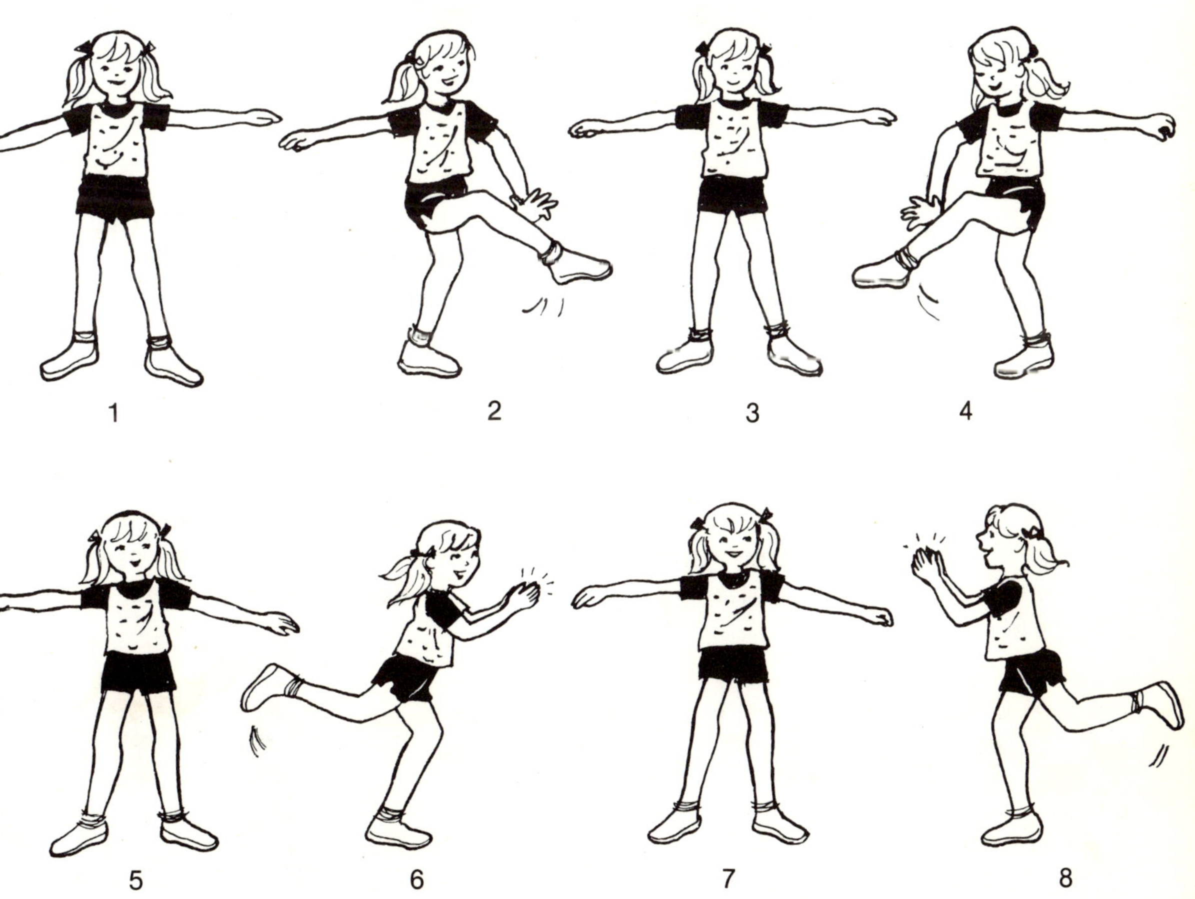

STEP 2

SIDE LOOKS

1. With left side to front, step left.
2. Swing right foot front.
3. Look back over left shoulder. Double-stomp left toes.
4. Look front. Double-stomp right toes.
5. Step left.
6. Swing right foot back.
7. Look back over left shoulder. Double-stomp left toes.
8. Look front. Double-stomp right toes.

Repeat Step 2.

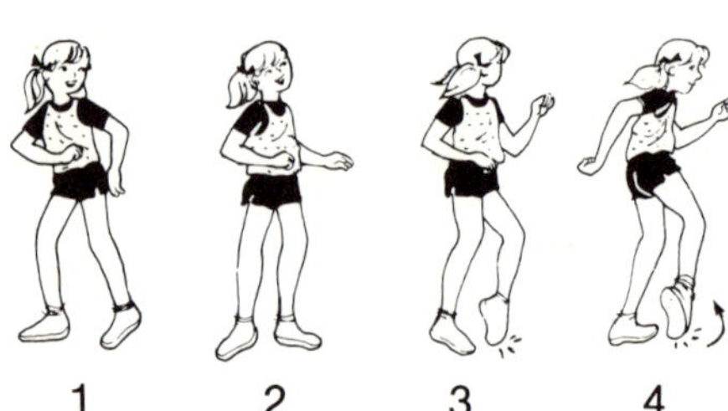

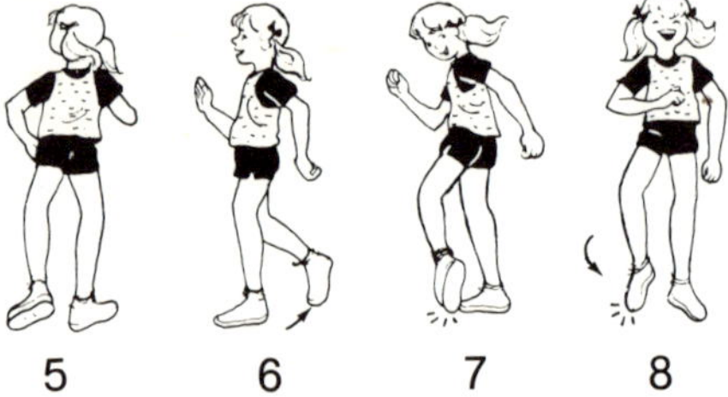

STEP 3

CAN-CANS

1. Feet apart, arms out at sides.
2. Lift right knee, then down.
3. Kick right leg front, then down. AST: Arms in front.
4. Lift left knee, then down. AST: Arms out.
5. Kick left leg front, then down. AST: Arms in front.
6. Lift right knee to side, then down. AST: Arms out.
7. Kick right leg to side, then down. AST: Arms in front.
8. Lift left knee to side, then down. AST: Arms out.
9. Kick left leg to side, then down. AST: Arms in front.

Repeat Step 3.

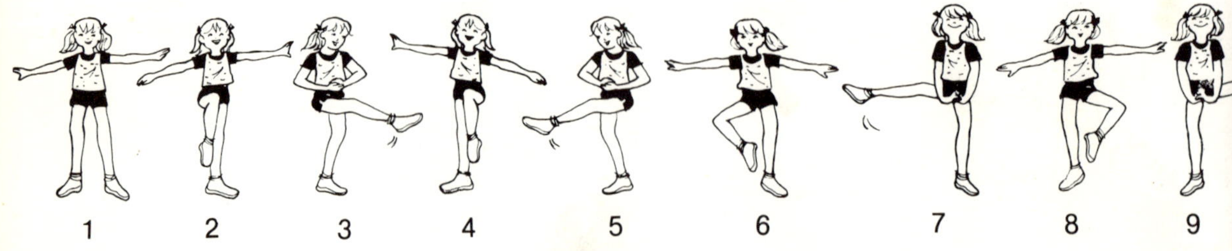

STEP 4

STEP-SLIDES

1. Step left. AST: Left arm out, right hand on right hip.
2. Slide right, closing feet together. AST: Clap hands.
3. Repeat 3 left Step-Slides.
4. Step right. AST: Right arm out, left hand on left hip.
5. Slide left, closing feet together. AST: Clap hands.
6. Repeat 3 right Step-Slides.

Repeat Step 4.

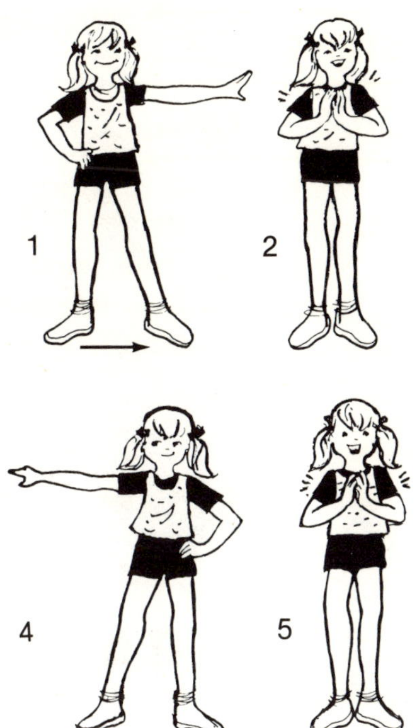

Repeat:
Step 1: Bend-Kicks
Step 2: Side-Looks
Step 3: Can-Cans
Step 4: Step-Slides
Step 1 (3 times), Step 2, Step 3 (1 time), Step 4, Step 1

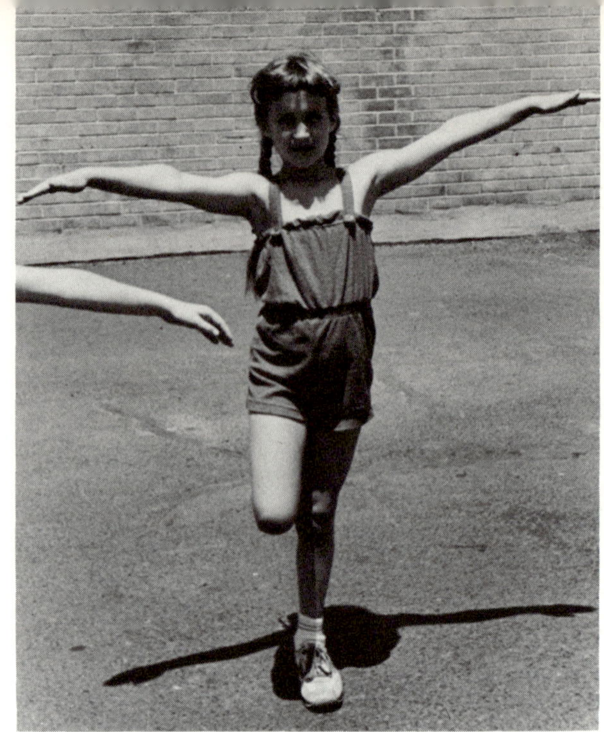

TANYA'S TICKLE

There are almost four minutes of twists, kicks, lunges, and fun in this next routine. Master the steps and then put as much oomph into each one as you can. You'll get a tickle out of the results!

Suggested music: *Let Me Tickle Your Fancy* (3:50 minutes), by Jermaine Jackson

Alternate music: *Planet Rock, Shake It Up*

INTRODUCTION:

Stand with feet apart, knees bent, arms bent at sides. Move up, down, up, down, up, down, up, down. (On each up movement, arms go out to sides.)

Repeat introduction.

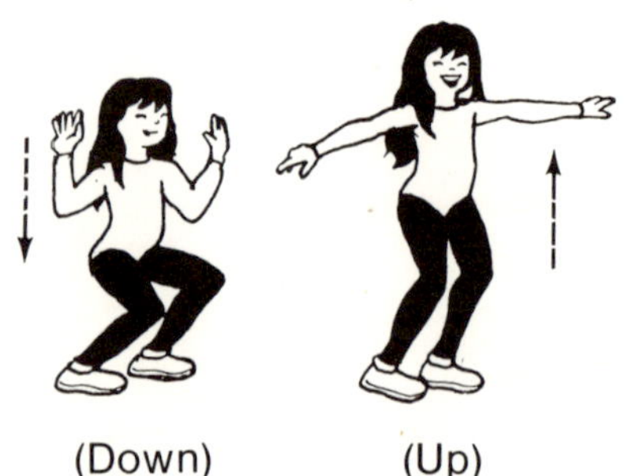

(Down) (Up)

STEP 1

HOP-LUNGES

1. Lunge right (left leg straight) and clap.
2. Hop-switch to lunge left (right leg straight) and clap.
3. Hop-switch to lunge right (left leg straight) and clap.
4. Hop-switch to lunge left (right leg straight) and clap.

Repeat Step 1.

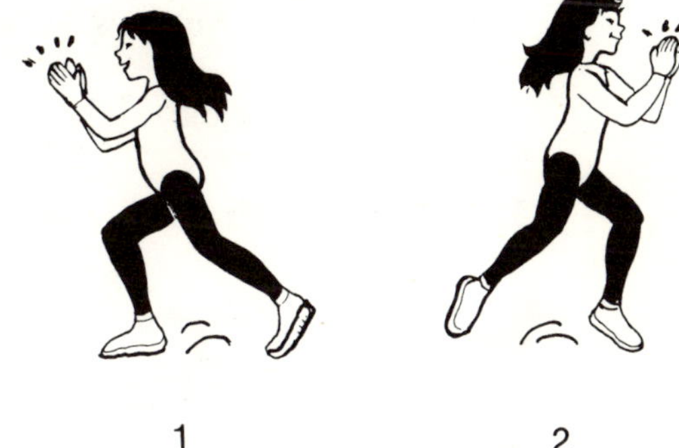

STEP 2

CROSS-KICKS

(Arms out at sides)

1. Move forward: Step right, left Cross-Kick.
2. Step left, right Cross-Kick.
3. Step right, left Cross-Kick.
4. Step left, right Cross-Kick.
5. Move backwards: Step right, left Cross-Kick.
6. Step left, right Cross-Kick.
7. Step right, left Cross-Kick.
8. Step left, right Cross-Kick.

Repeat Step 1 (Hop-Lunges)

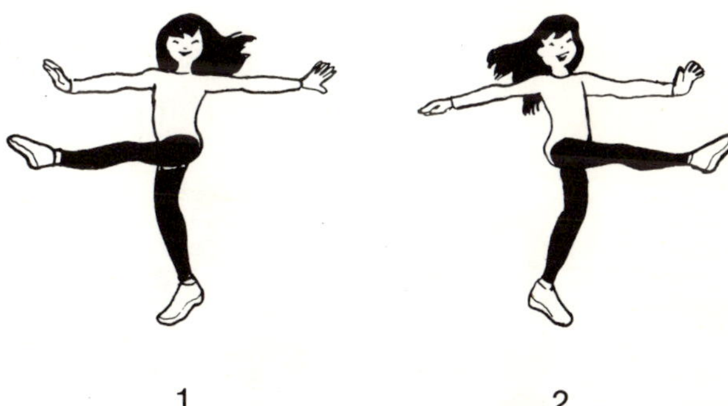

STEP 3

WIND-UPS

(Arms out at sides)
1. Step right, kick left leg back.
2. Step left, kick right leg back.
3. Step right, slide together.
4. Step right, kick left leg back.
5. Step left, kick right leg back.
6. Step right, kick left leg back.
7. Step left, slide together.
8. Step left, kick right leg back.

Repeat Step 3.

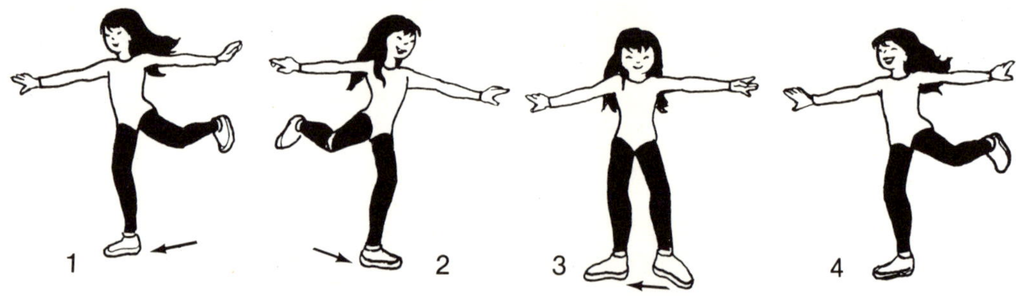

STEP 4

3-STEP TWIST

(Arms straight out)
1. Step forward: right, left, right.
2. Twist left knee across right leg.
3. Step back: left, right, left.
4. Twist right knee across left leg.

Repeat 3 times.

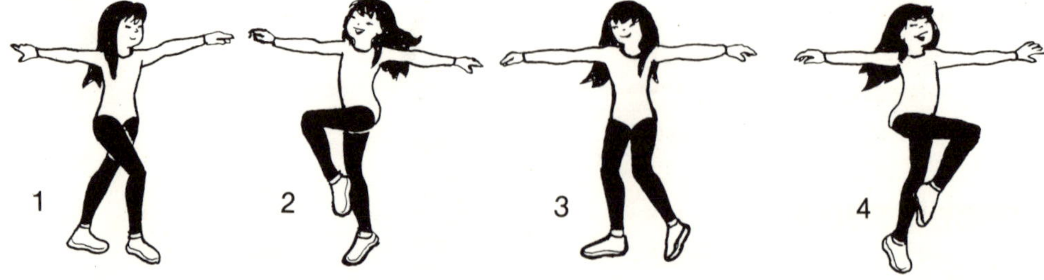

Repeat:
Step 3: Wind-Ups
Step 4: 3-Step-Twist
Step 2: Cross-Kicks
Step 1: Hop-Lunges

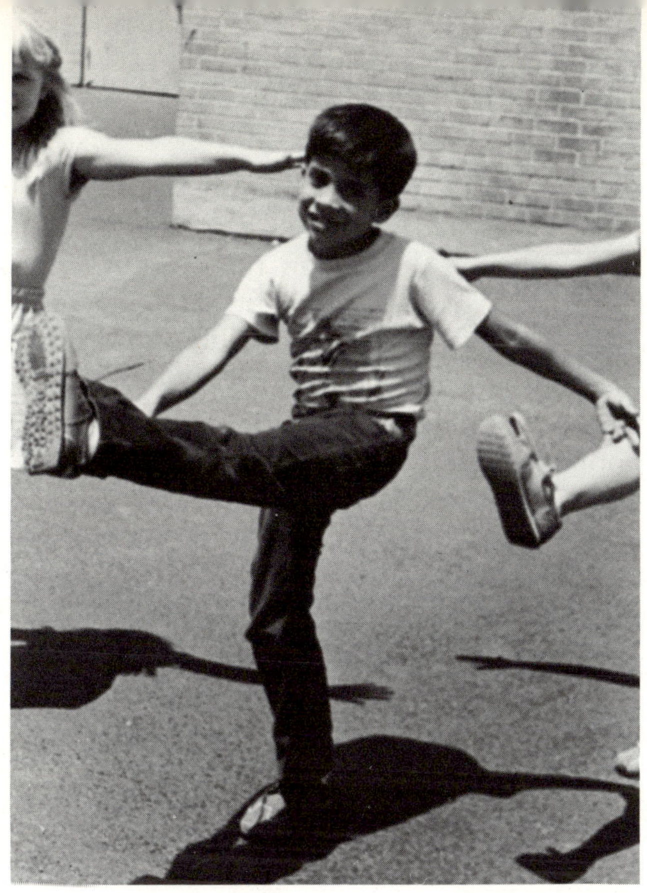

STEVIE'S SLIDE

We've set this peppy number to one of today's most popular releases. And when you let loose with it, Stevie's Slide should put a smile on your face and a little extra zing into your day.

Suggested music: *Mickey* (4:12 minutes), by Toni Basil
Alternate music: *Queen of Hearts*, by Bennie and the Jets

INTRODUCTION

Feet together, hands at sides. Bend/clap, straighten, bend/clap, straighten, bend/clap, straighten, bend/clap, straighten.

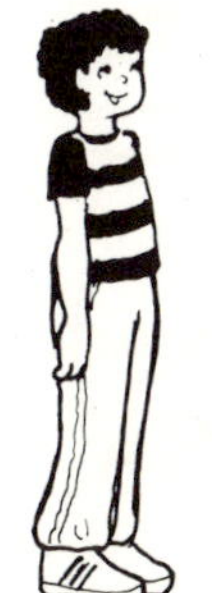

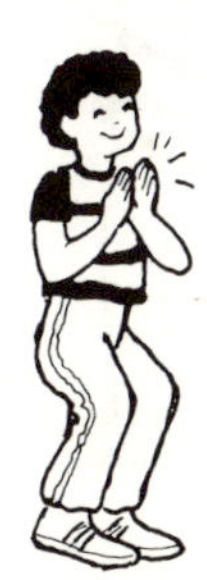

STEP 1

IN-PLACE RUNS

Start with left arm straight up, right arm straight out at side.
1. Run in place, turning left. AST: Bend both elbows in-out, in-out, in-out, in-out.
2. Run in place, turning right. Now right arm is straight up, left arm straight out at side. Bend elbows in-out, in-out, in-out, in-out.

Repeat Step 1.

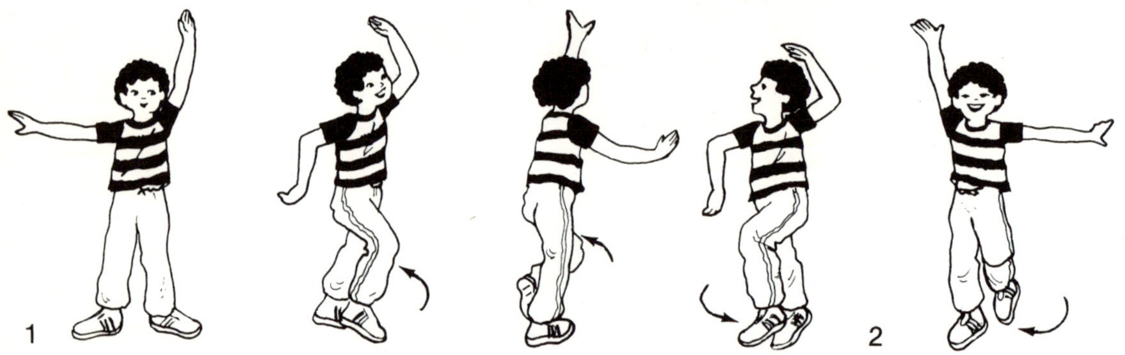

STEP 2

SIDE-CLAPS

(Hands out at sides "airplane angle")
1. Step right, slide right, closing feet together.
2. Step right, then clap.
3. Step left, slide left, closing feet together.
4. Step left, then clap.

Repeat step 3 times more.

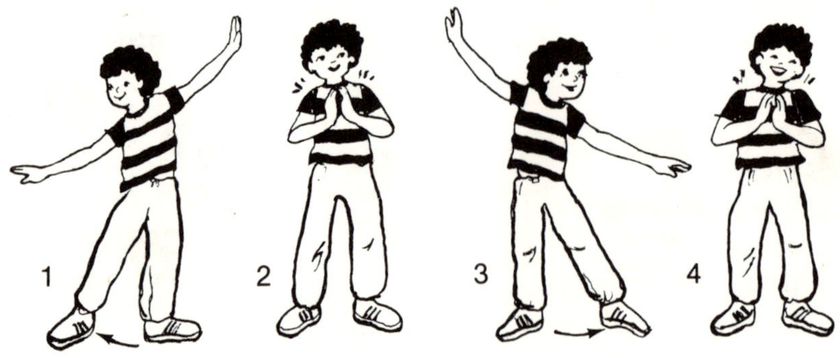

STEP 3

SWAY-TWISTS

1. Step right. AST: Sway arms over head to right.
2. Step left. AST: Sway arms over head to left.
3. Step right, sway right.
4. Step left, sway left, then drop arms to legs.
5. Twist left, right, left, right, left, right, left, right. AST: Arms move up.
6. Repeat Step 3.
7. Twist left, right, left, right.

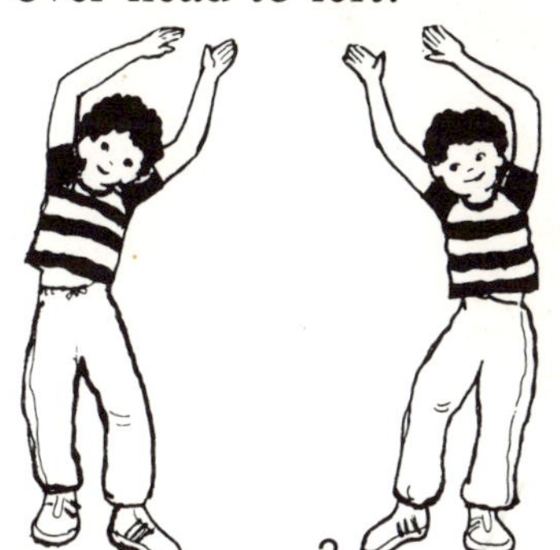

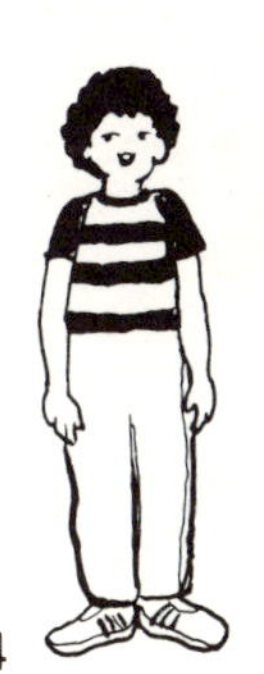

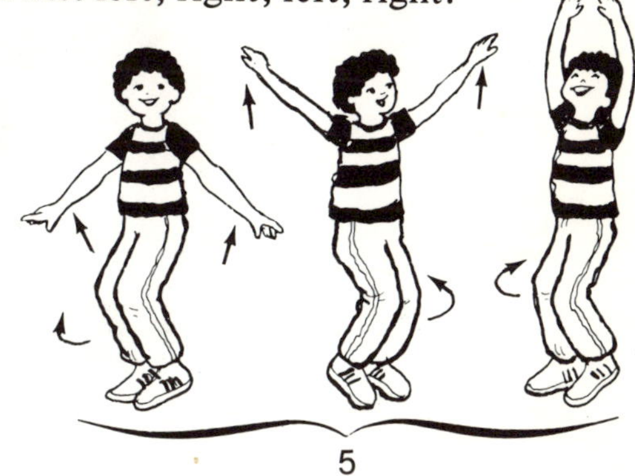

STEP 4

KNEE CROSS-LIFTS

1. Feet down, right hand on right hip.
2. Lift right knee across left leg and touch with left hand.
3. Right leg down.
4. Repeat right knee cross-lift 3 times (lift, down, lift, down, lift).

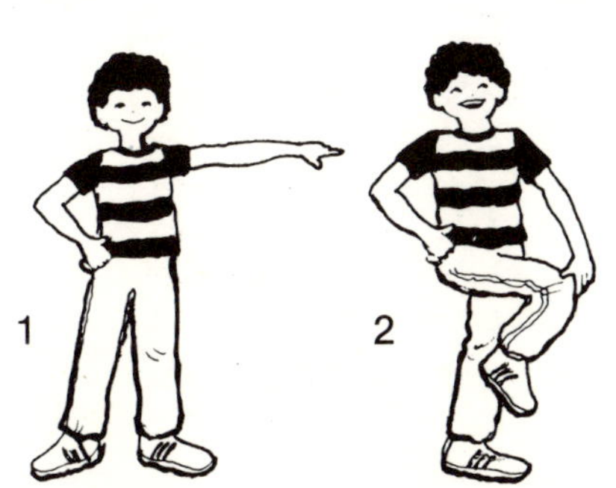

5. Feet down, left hand on left hip.
6. Lift left knee across right leg and touch with right hand.
7. Left leg down.
8. Repeat left knee cross-lift 3 times (lift, down, lift, down, lift).

Repeat Step 4.

Repeat:

Step 1: In-Place Runs
Step 2: Side-Claps
Step 3: Sway-Twists
Twist left, right, left, right.
Step 4: Knee Cross-Lifts
Twist left, right, left, right.
Step 1, Step 2, Step 3, Introduction, Step 1, Step 2, Twists, Step 4.

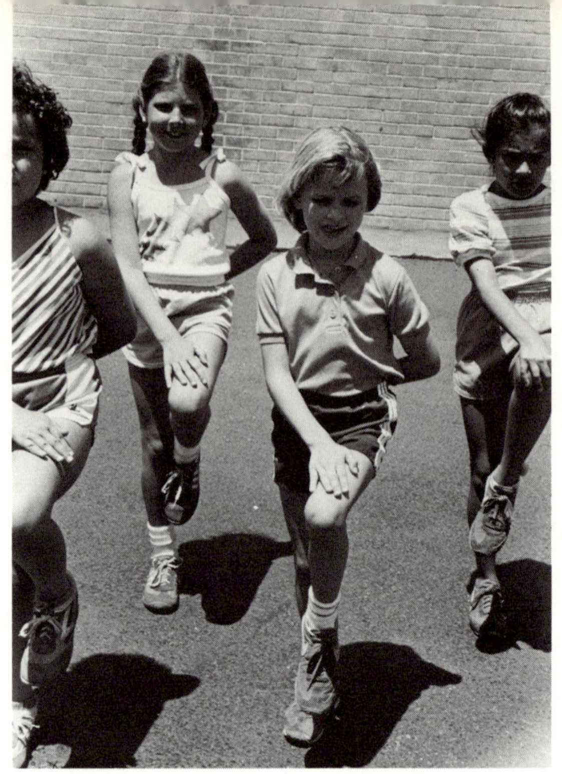

JANA'S JAZZ

Here's a happy snappy dance that puts you in the mood to celebrate simply being alive. Don't hesitate to shout out loud if you feel like it, and by all means have a good time!

Suggested music: *Celebration* (5:00 minutes), by Kool and the Gang
Alternate music: *Red Light* (from *Fame*)
Theme from *Shaft*

INTRODUCTION

KNEE-POPS

(Arms out at sides, knees slightly bent)
Right knee comes in-out. Left knee comes in-out. Right knee in-out, left knee in-out.

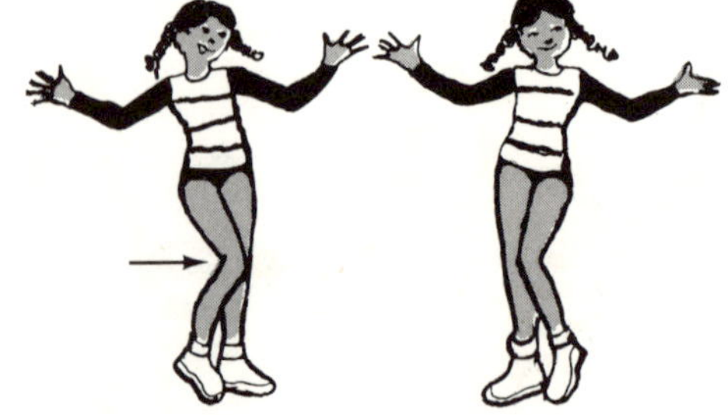

Repeat introduction.

STEP 1

SLIDE-SWINGS

1. Step right, closing feet together, right, together, right, together, right, together.
2. Swing hips right, left, right, left, right, left, right, left. AST: Clap hands.
3. Step left, closing feet together, left, together, left, together, left, together.
4. Swing hips left, right, left, right, left, right, left, right. AST: Clap hands.

Repeat Step 1.

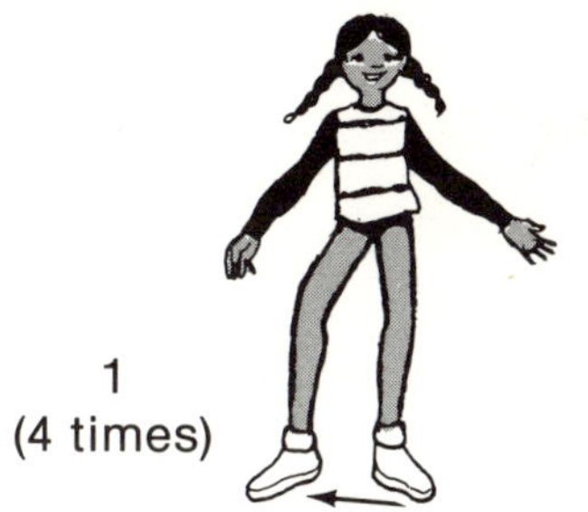
1 (4 times)

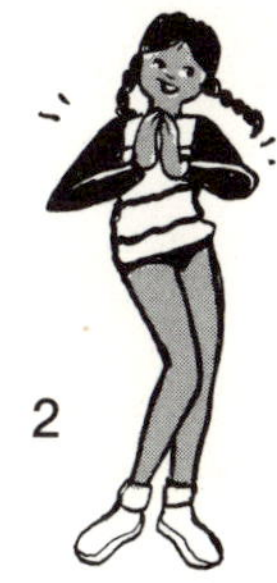
2

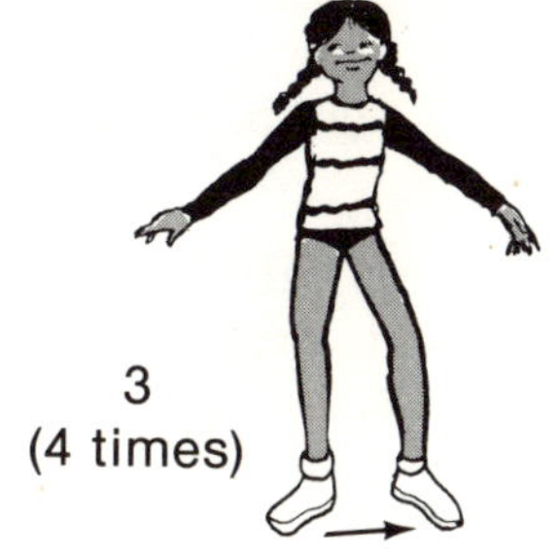
3 (4 times)

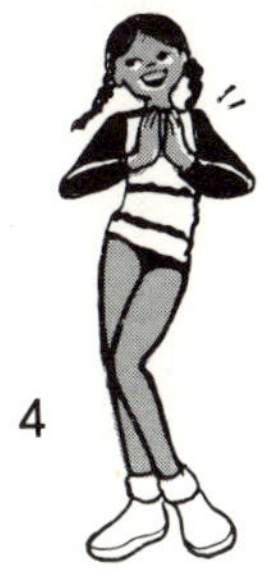
4

STEP 2

KICK-WALK

1. Stand with feet apart.
2. Kick left foot front. AST: Shrug shoulders.
3. Left foot down.
4. Kick right foot front. AST: Shrug shoulders.
5. Right foot down.
6. Kick left foot front. AST: Shrug shoulders.
7. Left foot down.
8. Kick right foot forward. AST: Shrug shoulders.
9. Slowly walk forward: Right toe-heel, left toe-heel, right toe-heel. (Swing arms as you move.)

Repeat Step 2.

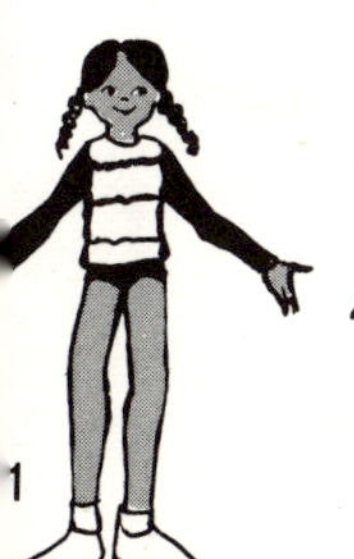
1

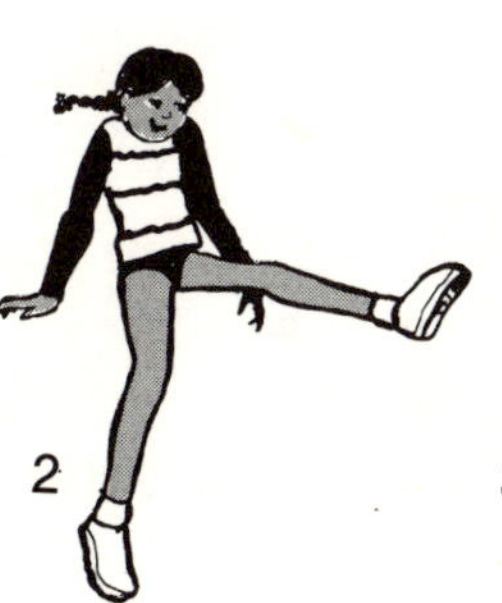
2

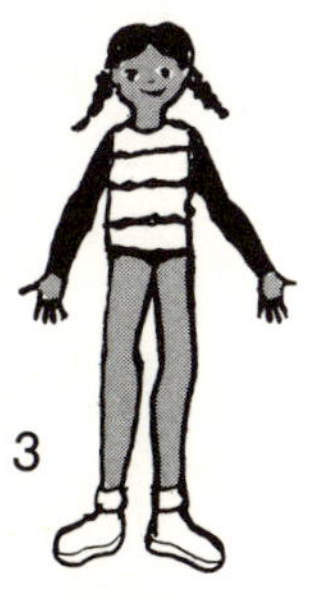
3

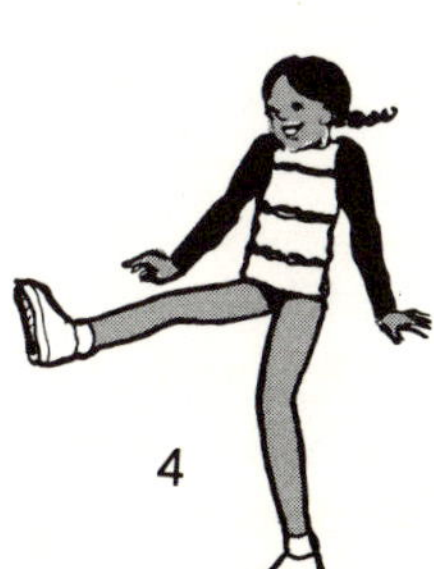
4

5 (Repeat of 1)
6 (Repeat of 2)
7 (Repeat of 3)
8 (Repeat of 4)

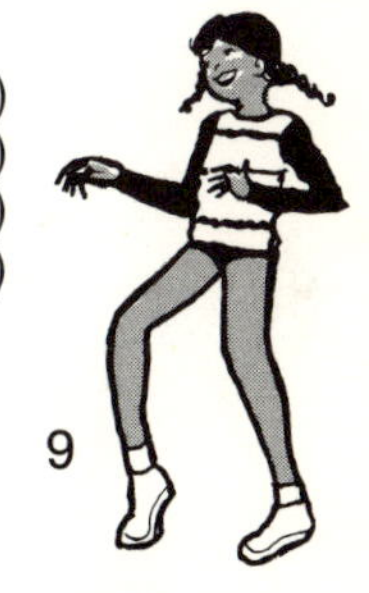
9

STEP 3

CROSS-WALKS

(Hand on hips)

1. Step right, cross left in front. Step right, cross left in back. Step right, cross left in front. Step right, cross left in back.
2. Step left, cross right in front. Step left, cross right in back. Step left, cross right in front. Step left, cross right in back.

Repeat Step 3.

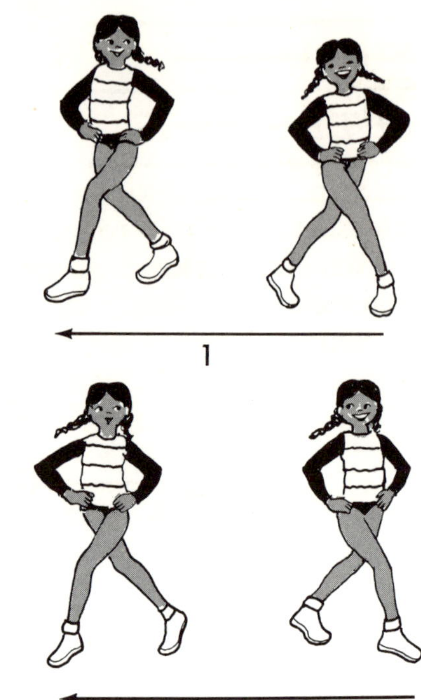

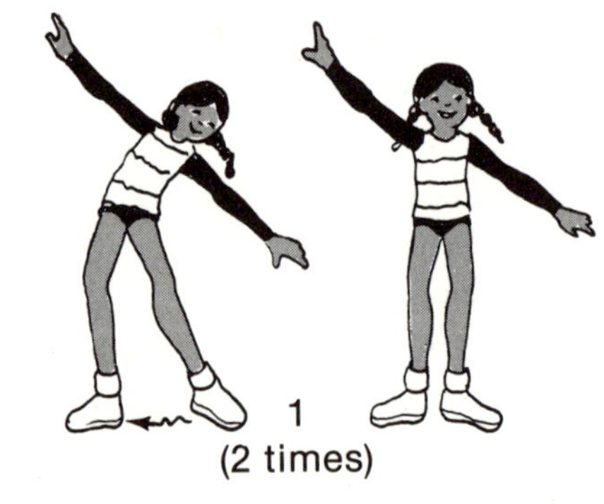

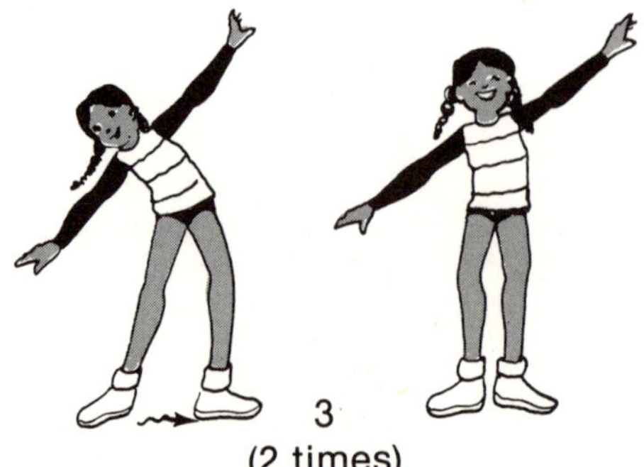

STEP 4

JAZZ LEANS

1. Step right, drag left foot to right foot. AST: right arm up, left arm down.
2. Repeat right Step-Drag
3. Step left, drag right foot to left foot. AST: left arm up, right arm down.
4. Repeat left Step-Drag

Repeat Step 4 three more times.

STEP 5

TURN-CLAPS

(Hands on hips)

1. Make a complete circle right; step right, left, right, clap.
2. Make a complete circle left; step left, right, left, clap.
3. Step front; right, left, right, clap.
4. Step back; left, right, left, clap.

Repeat Step 5.

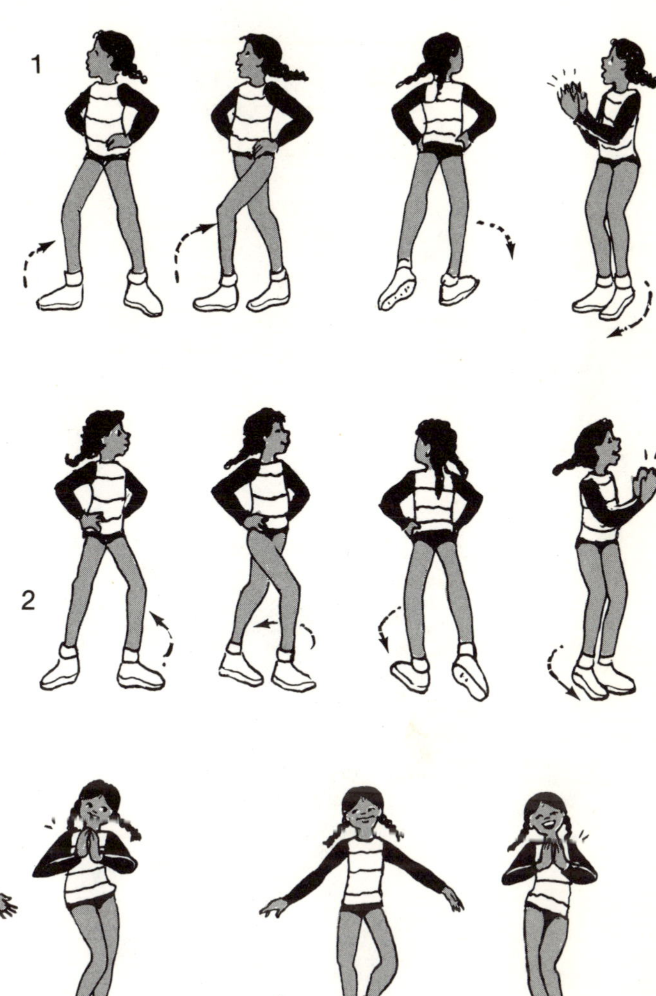

Repeat:
Step 1: Slide-Swings
Step 2: Kick-Walks
Step 3: Cross-Walks
Step 4: Jazz Leans
Step 5: Turn-Claps
Step 1, Step 2, Step 3, Step 5

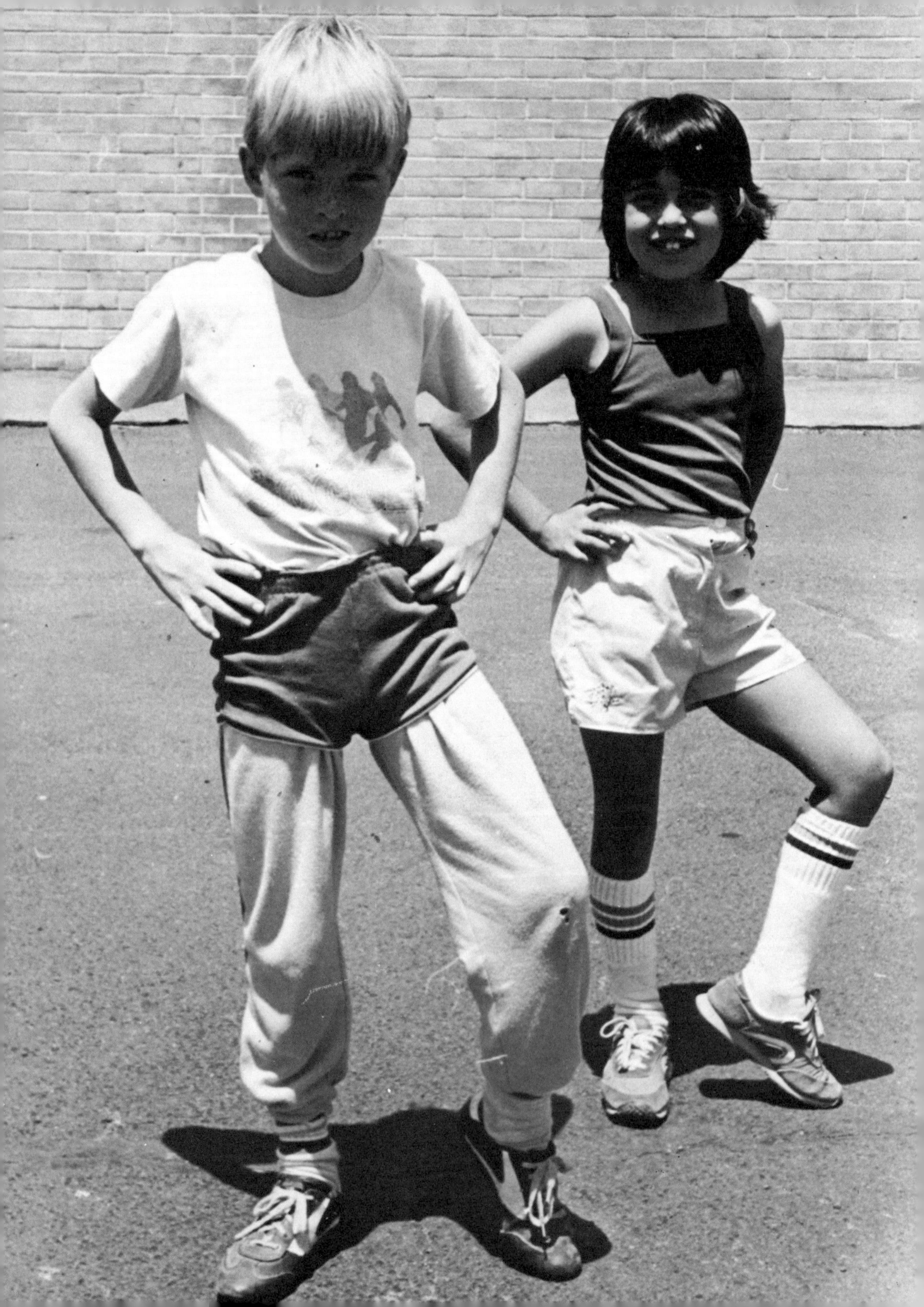

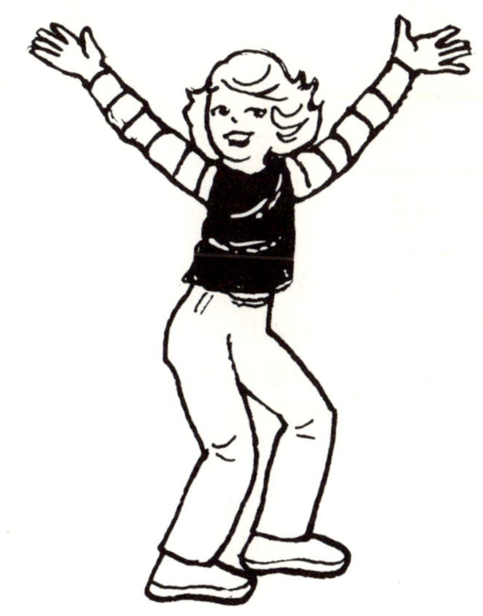

ROWENA'S ROCK

The last aerobics routine in your series of six, Rowena's Rock gives you plenty of room to jazz it up and use your imagination as your hands swing, your feet slide, and your whole body gets a head-to-toes workout.

Suggested music: *Fame* (5:14 minutes) from the soundtrack of the motion picture

Alternate music: *Our Love, Hello, Dolly*

INTRODUCTION

Stand with feet apart. Sway hips. Move arms up; cross left over right, right over left, left over right, right over left. Move arms down; cross right below left, left below right, right below left, left below right.

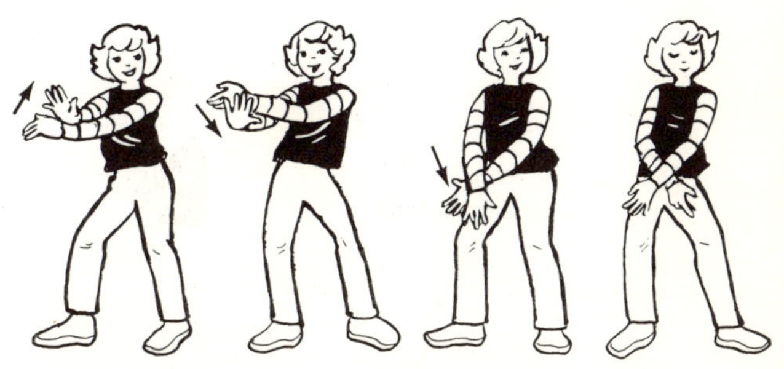

STEP 1

STEP-TOGETHER

(Hold hands above head)

1. Move right; step right, closing feet together, right, together, right, together, right, together.
2. Move left; step left, together, left, together, left, together, left, together.

Repeat Step 1.

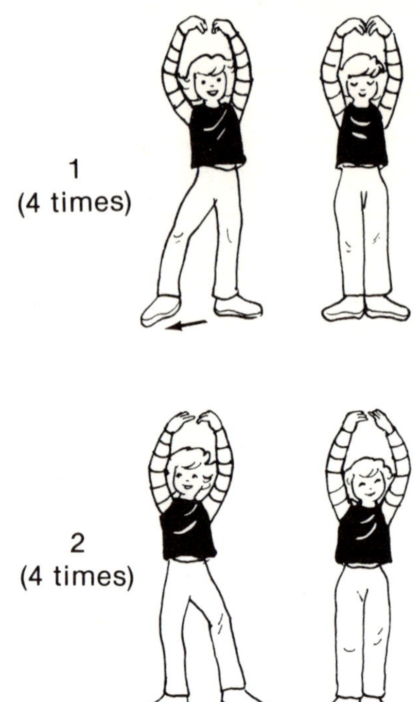

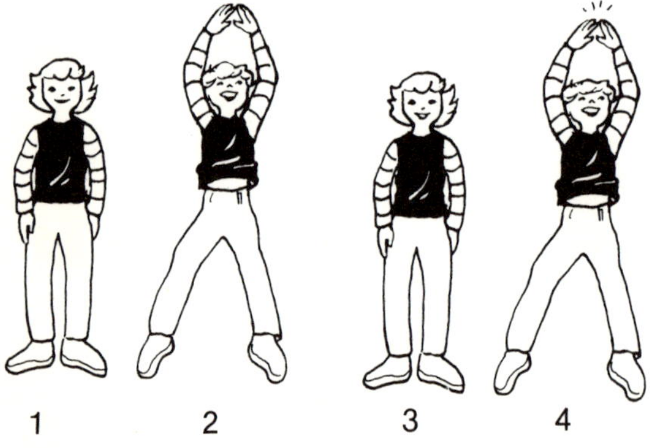

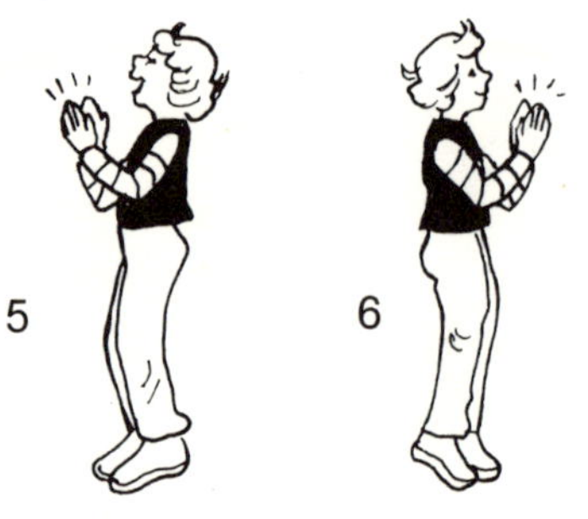

STEP 2

JUMPING JACKS

1. Face front, feet together, hands at sides.
2. Jump out. AST: Clap hands above head.
3. Jump close, hands at sides.
4. Jump out. AST: Clap hands above head.
5. Face right and clap.
6. Face left and clap.

Repeat Step 2 three more times.

STEP 3

DOUBLE WALKS

1. Walk right; right, left, right.
2. Step left back, left to side.
3. Step right back, right to side.
4. Step left back.
5. Walk left; left, right, left.
6. Step right back, right to side.
7. Step left back, left to side.
8. Step right back.

Repeat Step 3.

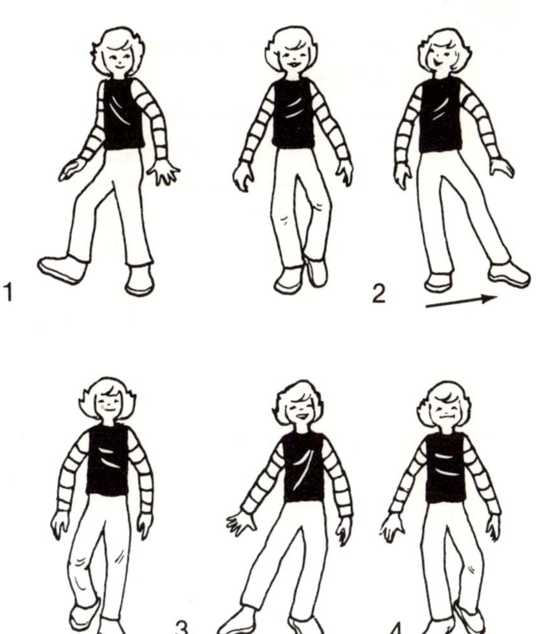

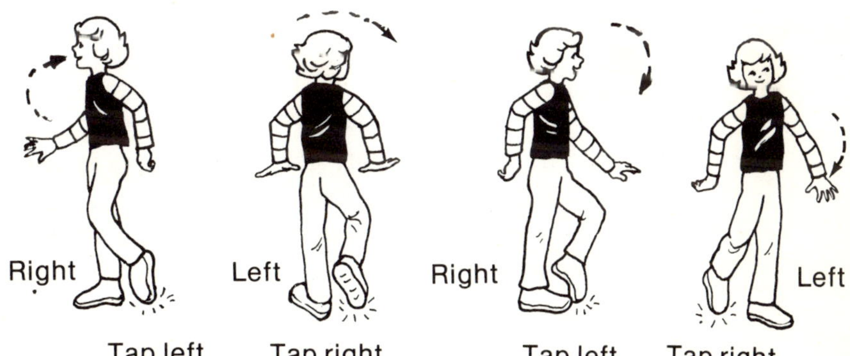

STEP 4

TOE-TAPS

1. Turn right; right, tap left, left, tap right, right, tap left, left, tap right.
2. Turn left; left, tap right, right, tap left, left, tap right, right, tap left.

Repeat Step 4.

STEP 5

SLIDE KNEE-BENDS

1. Step right, closing feet together, right, together, right, together, right.
2. Step left, right knee-bend.
3. Step right, left knee-bend.
4. Step left, together, left, together, left, together, left.
5. Step right, left knee-bend.
6. Step left, right knee-bend.

Repeat Step 5 three more times.

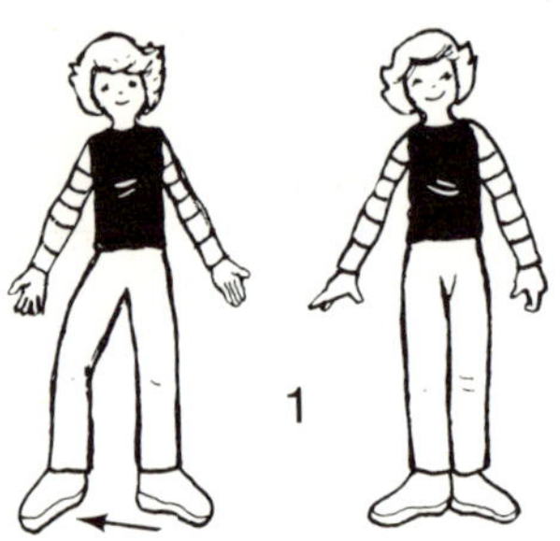

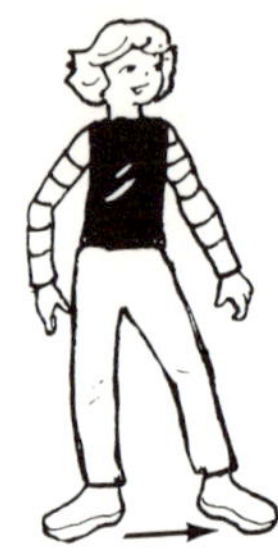

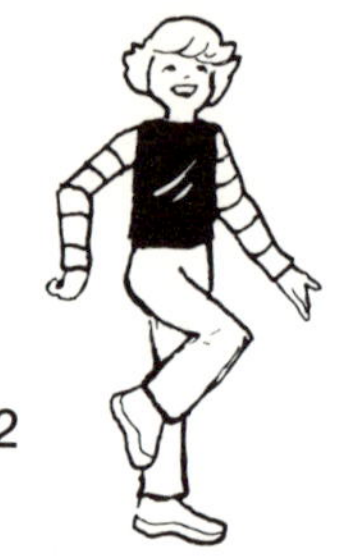

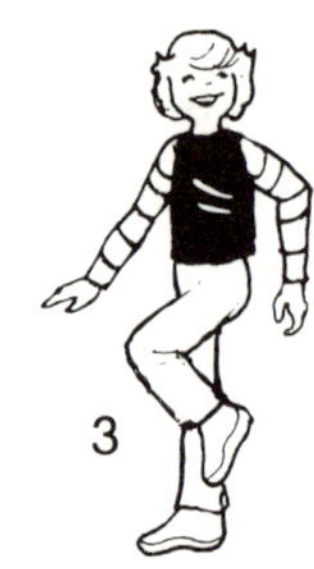

STEP 6

SQUIRMS

(Hands over head to start)

1. Squirm down; right, left, right, left, right, left, right, left. AST: Slowly lower arms.
2. Squirm up; right, left, right, left, right, left, right, left. AST: Slowly raise arms.

Repeat:

Step 1: Step-Together
Step 2: Jumping Jacks
Step 3: Double Walks
Step 5: Slide Knee-Bends
Step 4: Toe-Taps
Step 6: Squirms
Step 1, Step 2, Step 6, Step 5

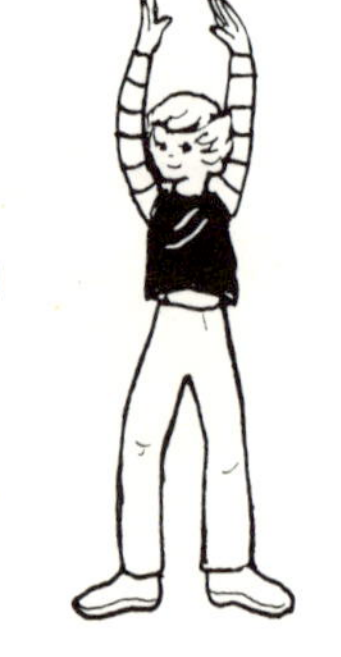

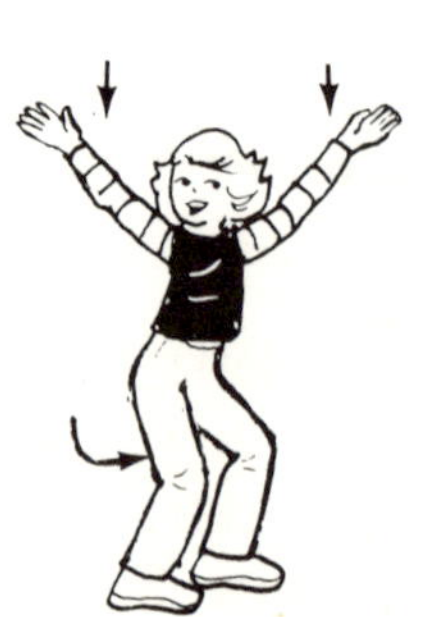

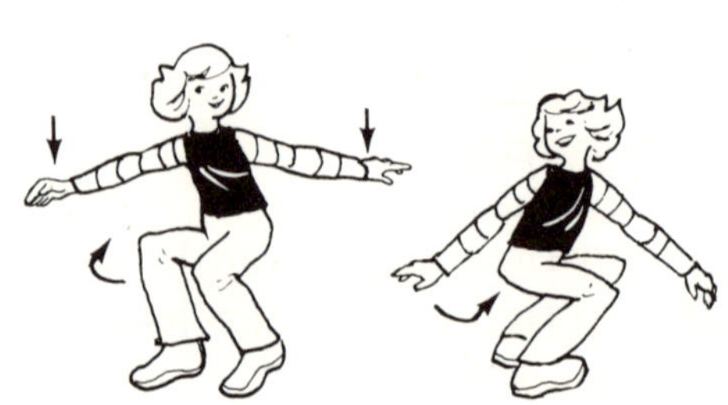

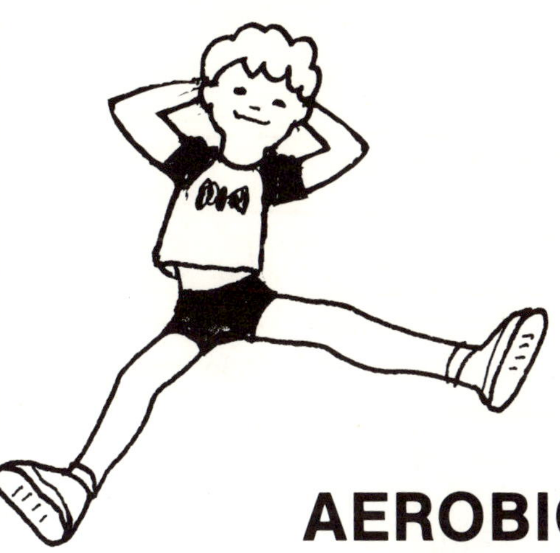

AEROBICS BASICS COOL-DOWNS

Cool-down exercises are an important part of your aerobic workout. They help your body readjust to normal activity after having gone through the rigors of your aerobic dances. Do each exercise slowly. Like your warm-up stretches, each cool-down should be held as you do a slow count of 5 (1000, 2000, 3000, 4000, 5000).

Suggested music: *Chariots of Fire*, by Vangelis,
Southern Nights, by Glen Campbell

COOL-DOWN 1

STANDING SWAY

A. Stand with your feet apart and both your hands over your head.
B. Sway your body to the right, then to the left. Do 5 times each side.

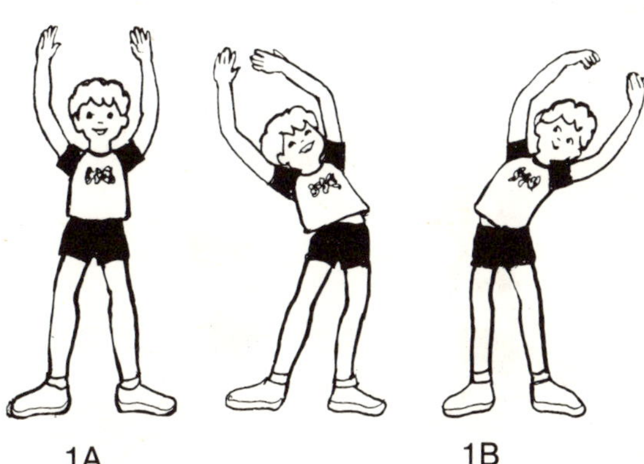

1A 1B

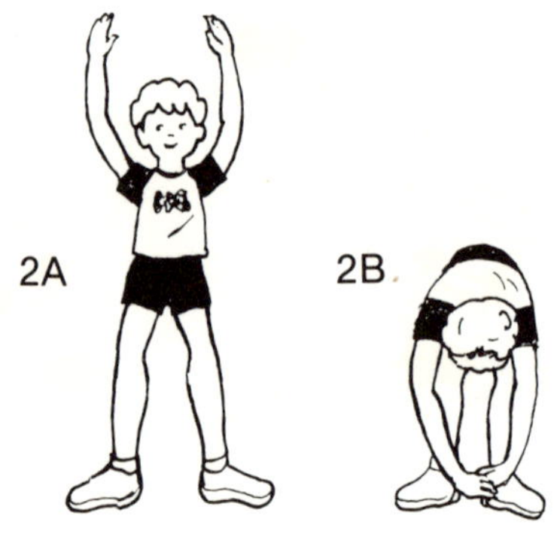

COOL-DOWN 2

CIRCLE-SWING

A. Start with feet slightly apart, hands in circle above your head.
B. Slowly bring your arms out and down and form a circle with hands together at your toes. Then extend hands out and circle again to starting pose.

Repeat 5 times.

COOL-DOWN 3

LIE-LIFT

A. Lie on floor with hands under head and legs together and up. Feet face forward.
B. Lower left leg to floor, then bring it back up. Lower right leg to floor, then bring it back up. Alternate lowering legs and raising them 5 times each.

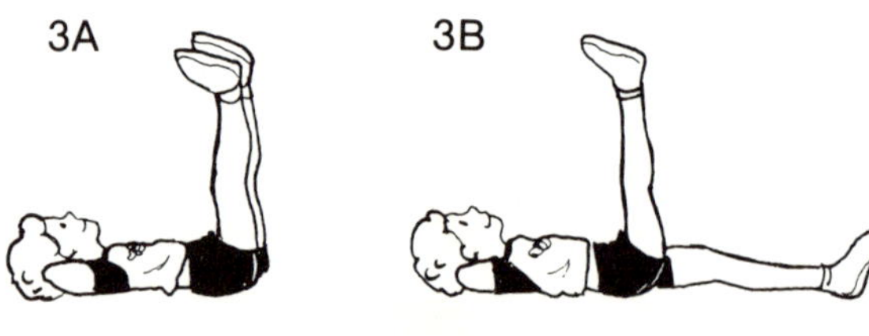

COOL-DOWN 4

SITTING STRETCH

A. Sit with feet spread apart, hands at sides.
B. Stretch arms out and up above head. Hold.
C. Return to original pose.

Repeat 5 times.

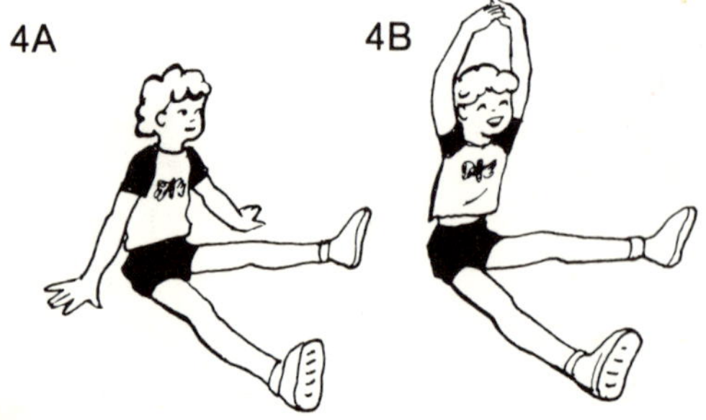

COOL-DOWN 5

SITTING BENDS

A. Sit on floor with hands behind head and feet apart.
B. Bend upper body to right.
C. Sit up straight again.
D. Bend upper body to left.
E. Sit up straight again.

Repeat 5 times.

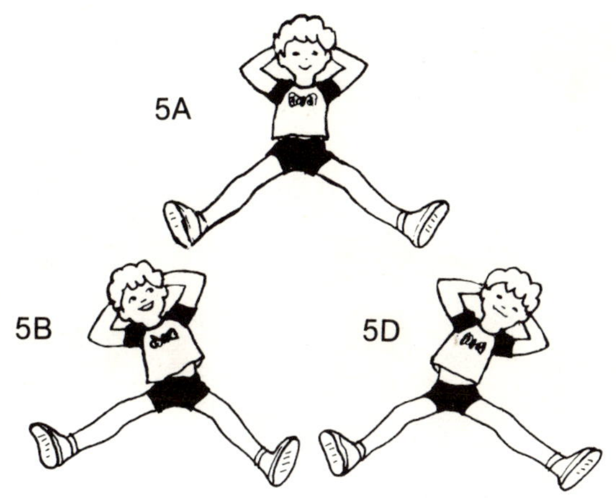

COOL-DOWN 6

SEATED TOE-TOUCH

A. Sit on floor with legs wide apart, hands at sides on floor.
B. Touch left foot with right hand, as left hand is extended back.
C. Return to *A* position.
D. Touch right foot with left hand, as right hand is extended back.
E. Return to *A* position.

Repeat 5 times.

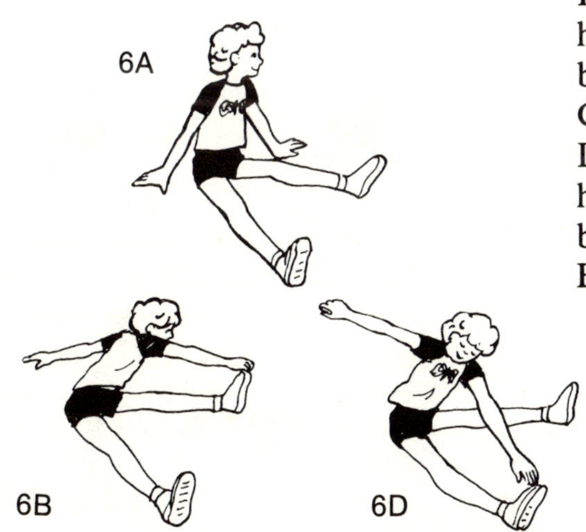

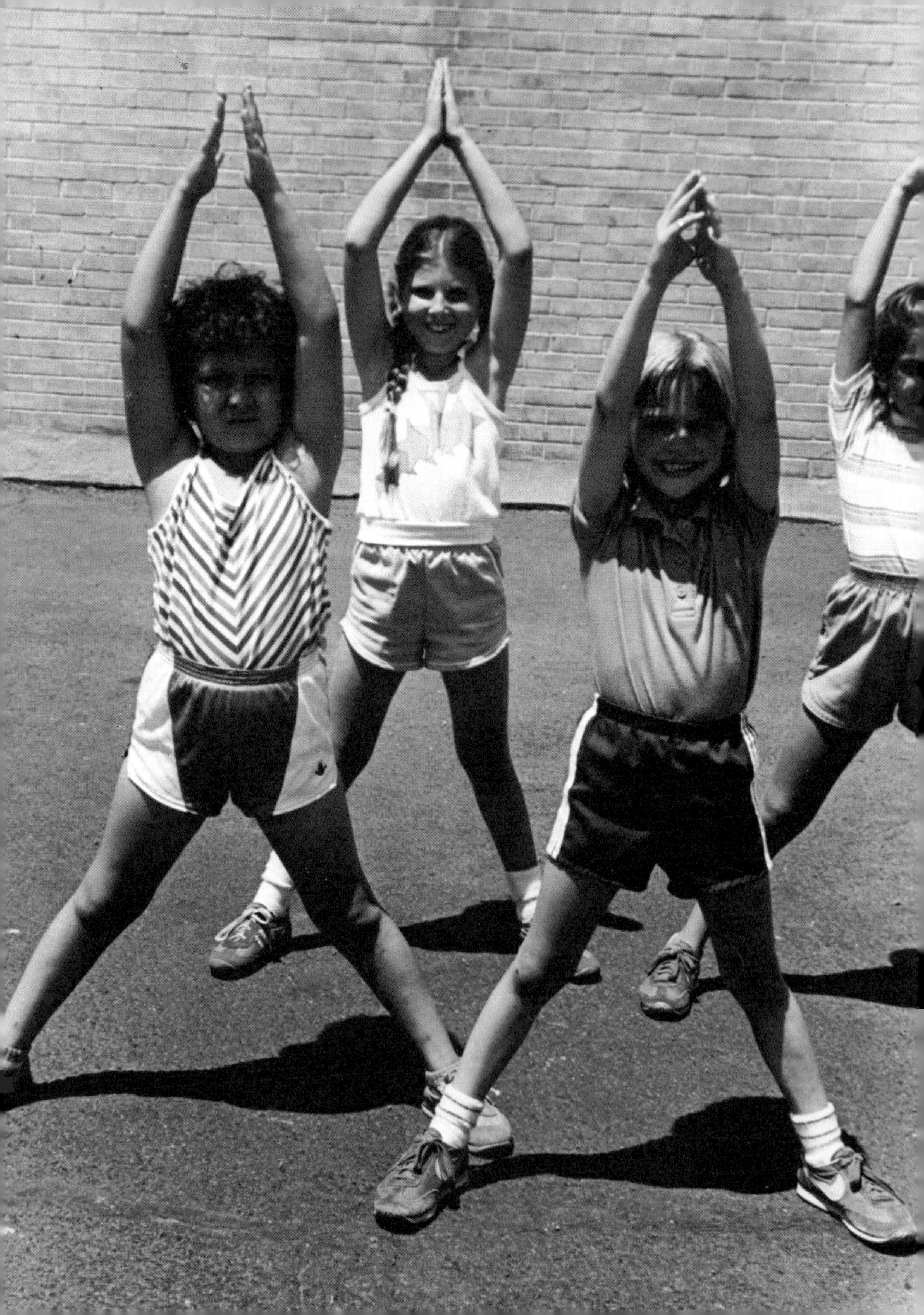

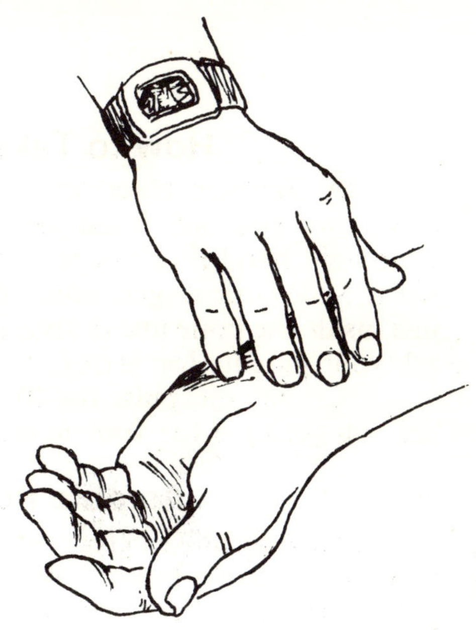

THE HEART OF AEROBICS

In order for an aerobics activity to be effective, you must do it continuously (usually for at least 15 minutes) and vigorously enough to raise your heart rate into what is called the "target zone."

To understand what this target zone is, you must first acquaint yourself with your maximum heart rate. This is the maximum number of times your heart beats per minute when your body is being maximally exerted. The maximum heart rate differs for different people, depending on their age, physical fitness, and size.

You can generally figure out your own maximum heart rate in beats per minute by subtracting your age from 220. If you are now 10 years old, your maximum heart rate will be 220 − 10 = 210.

Exercise physiologists urge people to do aerobic exercises that enable them to reach 70 to 85 percent of their maximum heart rate. And this is what is called their target zone.

At age 10, your target zone would be 70 to 85 percent of 210 or 147 to 178.5. You can discover whether you have reached your target zone by taking your pulse.

How to Take Your Pulse

A common place to check your pulse is on your wrist. First, turn your left hand palm up. Then place two fingers of your right hand (but not your thumb) over your upturned left wrist. Slide your fingers along until you feel your pulse beating just inside the bone under your left thumb. (If you have trouble, ask your parents for help.)

Count your pulse for 10 seconds. Then multiply the number you get by 6 for your heart beats per minute.

Aerobic Pulse-Taking

1. Check your pulse before you begin to exercise. This will give you your "resting pulse." When you were a baby, your resting pulse was somewhere between 130 to 150 beats per minute. At age 10, your pulse rate is approximately 70 to 100 beats per minute. And as an adult, your pulse rate will be approximately 60 to 80 beats per minute. (However, the more exercise you do, the lower your resting rate will become. Some athletes who are in excellent condition have resting pulses as low as 35 to 45 beats per minute!)

2. At various intervals during your aerobic activity period check your pulse. Don't stop but jog or walk in place. See if you are in your target zone. If you are above that zone, you may want to exercise *less* vigorously. If you are below that zone, you may want to exercise *more* vigorously.

3. Check your pulse five minutes after you have finished exercising. The better the shape you are in, the faster your pulse will return to its resting rate.

You can score yourself "fit as a fiddle" when your pulse takes less than 45 seconds to return to its resting rate after a 5 to 10 minute aerobic workout.

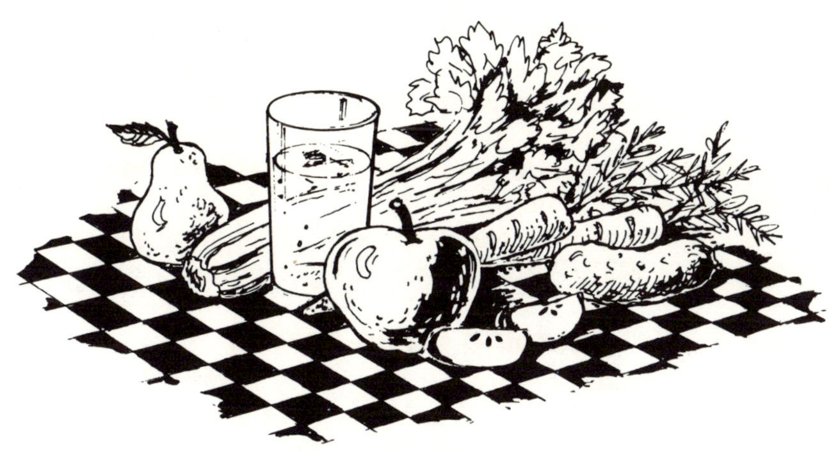

FOOD FOR THOUGHT

While regular exercise is vital to your well-being, it is only part of the total picture. Food is another major influence on your health and your appearance.

Nutritionally good foods help you feel good and look good as well. Nutritionally bad foods, on the other hand, destroy complexions, damage teeth, and ruin shapes and dispositions.

The biggest culprit is junk food—those easy-to-eat snacks we grab on the run or mindlessly munch while watching our favorite shows on TV. They may taste yummy in the short run, but in the long run they can cause trouble we then have to spend money and/or time to correct.

Junk foods are often high in calories, too. Calories represent the amount of energy—or heat—each food we eat produces. Calories—or energy—not immediately used up in our basic bodily functions or muscular activities get stored as fat. And if you keep supplying your body with more calories than your activities require, your fat reserve and you grow larger . . . and larger . . . and larger.

The following are some good snacks to replace bad ones. Notice that the good snacks are lower in calories, as well as higher in nutritional value.

COMPARE THE CALORIES . . . MAKE YOUR CHOICE

MENU A	MENU B
Apple (medium) 58	Apple pie (1 piece) 346
Applesauce (¼ cup) 52	Milkshake 400
Broccoli - 1 stalk 45	Banana Split 400
Carrots (raw) 1 cup 20	Cupcake (1) 130
Celery (1 piece) 2	Potato Chips (10) 100
Cucumber (1) 30	Chocolate candy (1) 150
Pears, (fresh) (1 medium) 100	Pears, canned (1 cup) 195

Here are some hints to help you and your family eat more nutritionally. Perhaps you will want to make some changes in the way you eat today.

1. Don't eat when you are upset. Sometimes when we are yelled at, or are upset for some reason, we seek comfort by filling our mouths. But eating won't make a problem go away. And it may add extra pounds that will give us yet another worry!

2. Think twice before you pour gobs of high caloric gravies on meats or salad dressings on salads. Just a teaspoonful is often enough. A smart idea is to always have gravies and dressings served in a separate bowl, so you can take as much or as little as you want.

3. Drink water! Water is great for cleaning out your system. Besides, it has no calories or sugar.

4. Eat slowly. Really taste and digest each spoonful or forkful of food you take.

5. Go easy on salt. Salt is a major hazard for people who suffer from high blood pressure. It is a good idea to start cultivating a taste for foods without salt as early as possible in life. (Lots of herbs and seasonings make great substitutes.)

6. Voice your preferences! Ask to have more healthy snacks and foods in your house. The more good choices you have around, the more likely you are to snack right and enjoy more nutritious meals.

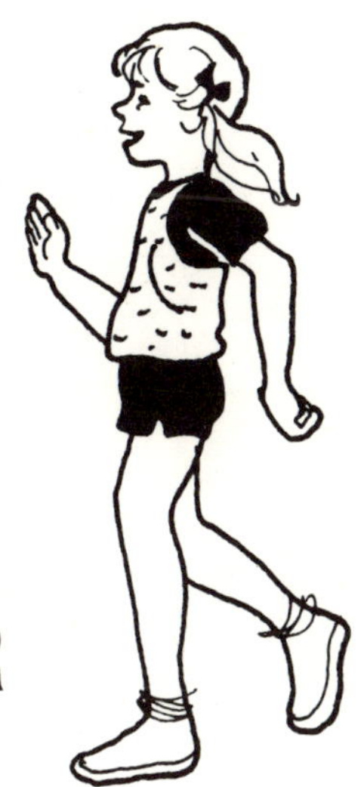

ACTIVATING YOUR EVERY DAY

As you learned earlier, many activities can be aerobic as long as your pulse rate reaches its target zone. Basketball, biking, folk dancing, hiking, skating, cross-country skiing, swimming—even playing tag and walking briskly can be aerobic.

Chances are you're already naturally active. You run around a lot just getting from here to there. But you may be like many children today who are TV addicts, or you may be a confirmed bookworm. In either case, you may spend more time watching or reading than you do moving around.

If you feel a bit less active than you know you should be, aerobic dancing is a fantastic way to start changing your everyday habits.

And here are just a few additional suggestions to add some steps to your life.

1. Whenever you go someplace where there is an escalator or elevator, opt for the stairs instead. (Chances are, you'll beat the escalator up anyway.)

2. Walk instead of riding whenever possible. Perhaps you can persuade a group of friends to walk to school together in the morning. A biking group is another idea. You might team up with a friend, or group of friends, and bike once or twice a week.

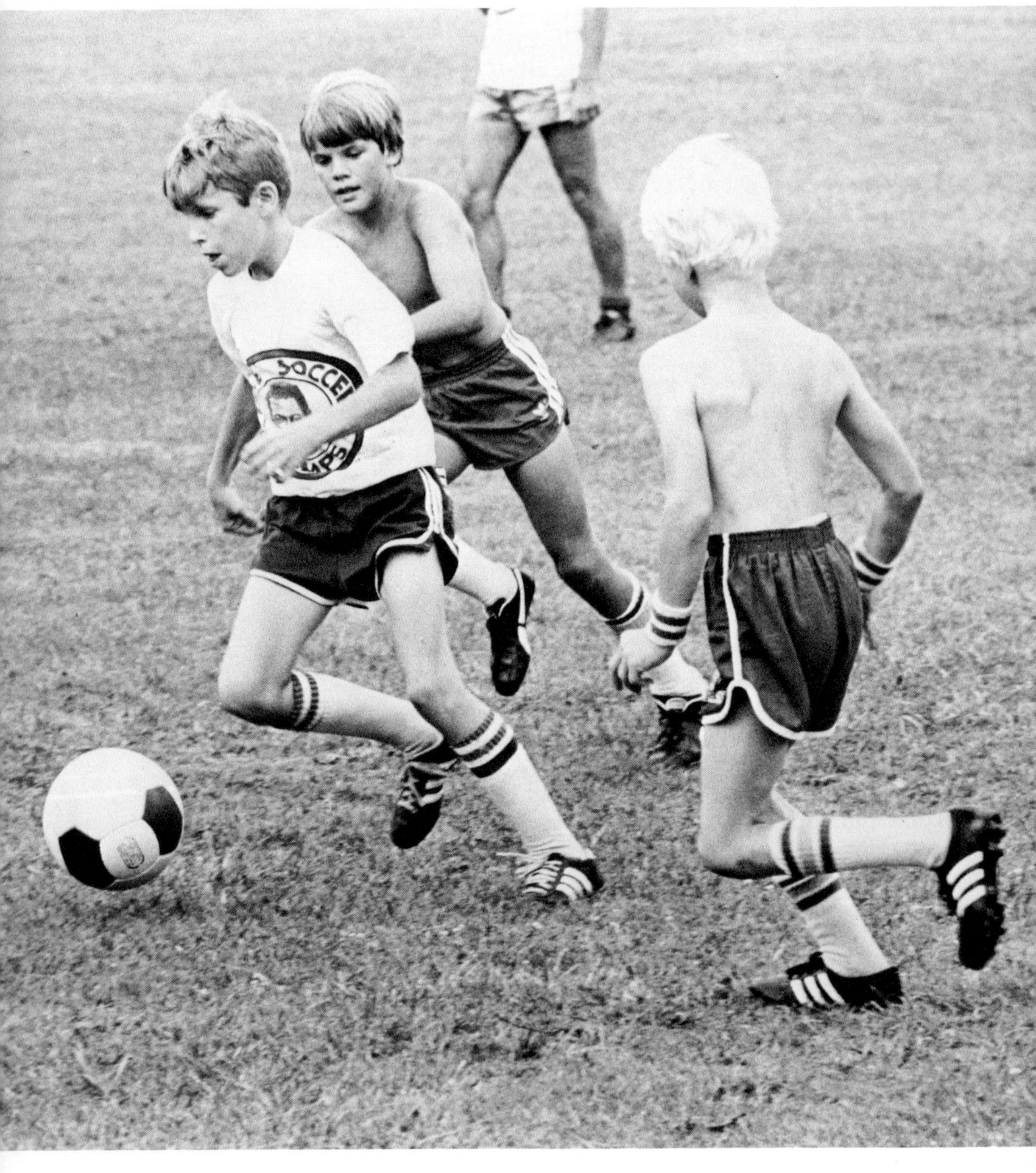

3. Find a sport you like. Bookworms, especially, need to be reminded that sports can be fun. Besides, being active actually helps you think better. And if you have a sticky problem to solve, you will be surprised at how getting involved in an activity actually helps you solve it faster! (Because your mind often clicks away subconsciously, you get your exercise and the problem gets solved as well!)

And there are so many wonderful sports to choose from; swimming or soccer or tennis are three possibilities. Find a friend or relative who is active in a sport that interests you and ask if he or she is willing to show you how to play the game.

4. Say yes to errands. You are probably asked to do things older people find difficult to do. "You're young," they'll say. "Run upstairs and get my glasses." Instead of making a face, do such tasks happily. Those extra efforts you make every day will turn out to be for your own good.

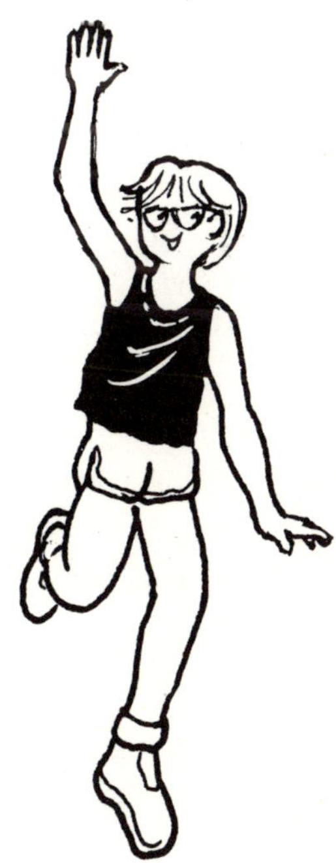

INDEX